WORST FEAR:

*One Woman's Story of
Brain Surgery and Survival*

TONI FERRUCCI
WITH CHRISTOPHER GILSON

Copyright ©1997 by Toni Ferrucci

Published by Rising Star Publications, Inc.
353 High Street
Closter, NJ 07624

Printed in the United States of America

First Printing

ISBN 1-888770-03-1

To Richard, my husband,
whose love gave me the strength
I needed to survive.

Foreword

Brain tumors continue to be one of the most dreaded diagnoses in medicine, for patients, families, and physicians alike. Indeed, the incidence of primary central nervous system tumors is currently about 6.5 malignant (i.e. cancerous) and an additional 10 benign brain tumors per 100,000 adults each year. However, this number is rising; this year 17,500 adult Americans will be diagnosed with primary brain tumors – those arising from the brain and its coverings. And close to 100,000 people will develop metastatic brain tumors – those arising elsewhere in the body and spreading to the brain.

Although overall mortality from these tumors has also increased, this rise has not paralleled the change in incidence. That is, data from the National Cancer Institute's Surveillance, Epidemiology, and End Results (SEER) Program have demonstrated a significant improvement in survival from malignant brain tumors, or cancers, during the late 1980s for both men and women. While the National Cancer Institute's objective of a 50 percent reduction in all cancer mortality by the year 2000 will not be realized, for the first time advances in the laboratory and in the clinic are contributing to longer and happier lives for individuals with brain tumors. Refinements in magnetic resonance imaging (MRI), microsurgery, radiosurgery, gene therapy, implantable chemotherapy, and treatments with biologic response modifiers will likely yield another generation of advances. Brain tumor patients are becoming survivors.

Toni Ferrucci is one of these survivors. Fortunately for us, she has had the courage to put to paper what others have feared to talk about, or feared to ask, or feared to think. In this book she details her odyssey with her own brain tumor from the first vague symptoms, to diagnosis, to treatment, to her ongoing daily life. She brings us her emotions and thoughts during each step of her ordeal, while providing understandable explanations of tests, procedures, and therapies encountered by nearly all brain tumor patients. Her end of chapter *"Reflections"* provide particularly good insights and approaches to issues that all brain tumor patients will encounter.

Patients with brain tumors are certainly a heterogeneous lot: with benign tumors such as meningiomas, pituitary adenomas, acoustic neuromas, craniopharyngiomas, gangliogliomas, hemangioblastomas; and malignant tumors such as astrocytomas (sometimes referred to as gliomas), oligodendrogliomas, ependymomas, lymphomas, and metastases. No one explanation can answer every conceivable question. Nevertheless, with her interpretations, Ms. Ferrucci finds a common denominator of prerequisite information for all brain tumor patients and their families.

Brain tumors and the field of neuro-oncology tend to be all too unique a domain for a small group of physicians, who often provide wonderful care and direction but lack the perspective of the patient. Neurosurgeons, neurologists, and oncologists can expertly explain the physiologic barriers separating the nervous system from the rest of the body, or the inability of a damaged nervous system to regenerate in a meaningful fashion, or the heterogeneity of symptoms referable to various anatomic locations within the brain. These same physicians cannot, however, convey the day-to-day thoughts or emotions experienced by the patient who has the tumor. With her remarkable story, Ms. Ferrucci's first-person narrative picks up where the physician stops.

Worst Fear is a welcome addition to neuro-oncology for patients, families, friends, and even physicians. Ms. Ferrucci's story not only improves our awareness, but is also another step in changing brain tumors and their treatment from a pattern of failure to a pattern of success. With a unique combination of information and optimism, Ms. Ferrucci has successfully conquered her worst fear as many more individuals will continue to do with her help.

The future successes of neuro-oncology will depend on the continuing research, but optimism such as Toni Ferrucci's will be an essential ingredient for all survivors.

Paul Graham Fisher, M.D., M.H.S.
Assistant Professor
Departments of Neurology,
    Oncology, and Pediatrics
The Johns Hopkins University
    School of Medicine
Baltimore, Maryland

Preface

The long journey with brain tumor surgery that began for me in the summer of 1991 has prompted many questions about my experience. Questions that might help others facing or recovering from such surgery. For this reason, medical people and patients alike have encouraged me to write my story.

In writing it, I realize how impossible it would have been to survive my series of often anxious and critical experiences without learning some things that can be of benefit not only to patients, but to those close to them. Since this learning process continued at every stage along the way, relevant observations and comments are included at the end of each chapter. In a number of cases, these are addressed to family members and friends, as well as to patients. I sincerely hope that they will be of as much value to others as they would have been to me.

Acknowledgements

Thanks and love go to my children Lee, Michael, Susan, and Richard II, who were brave and tremendously encouraging through the darkest time.

Deep thanks and appreciation go to Christopher Gilson, who co-authored this book with me and whose patience and thoroughness made my job easy.

To Estelle Lee, my mother, for endless hours of reading and typing the chapters to be sure they were just the way they should be; and to my sister Maryann Daly who, among the countless other things she did for me, finally got the computer to do what we wanted.

And my heartfelt thanks for all the friends who were always there to help in ever so many ways, as well as to the wonderful doctors, technicians, assistants, nurses, and therapists whose care and skills brought me safely through my long, perilous medical journey.

Introduction

Shattering news comes to Toni Ferrucci, 44, of Garden City, New York, in a Friday-afternoon telephone call late in June of 1991. An MRI has revealed that recurring neck aches and episodes of disorientation are due to a large, dangerous tumor in her brain. An operation is imperative.

At first devastated, she regains her composure and rationalizes that other individuals have faced and survived brain surgery. She resolves to be positive and take the whole thing in stride.

In viewing the MRI pictures, she and her husband Richard learn how difficult and delicate the operation will be. The tumor, lemon-sized, is in a highly vulnerable location on the stem at the base of her brain. Extreme caution will be needed to avoid injuring the vital nerves that serve as highways for messages from the brain to the body.

Thus begins in the fall of 1991 a long medical journey that takes her first to New York Hospital for what turns out to be but an initial operation. Despite nine solid hours of effort, only a relatively small portion of the tumor has been removed.

The tumor, however, is a slow-growing type. Although another operation is in prospect, what has been done to the growth tissue may postpone further surgery for a while. Periodic MRIs will tell.

Meanwhile, there are lingering aftereffects from the surgery itself and the medications it required: Double vision in the right eye. Paralysis in the right side of the face. "Moon syndrome" – puffed face and blimp-like body. Weird spaced-out sensations that come with no warning and create extreme anxiety. Diminished attention span and frustrating memory lapses. An insatiable craving for sweets.

With the help of family and friends and through her own determination, Toni learns to cope with these persistent aftermaths and progressively surmounts them.

As a result, except for having to compensate for continuing double vision and right-side facial paralysis, she is able to resume a normal life. This holds until late in 1993. It is then that an MRI shows definite tumor growth and she begins experiencing obvious symptoms that pressure on the brain has returned.

A brain-tumor-related article in *Reader's Digest* leads her early in 1994 to the George Washington University Medical Center in Washington, D.C. She goes there to see one of five surgeons in the world who have gained reputations for successful operations on brainstem tumors in adults.

The operation that follows is in two stages, consumes 22 hours, and succeeds in removing 75-80 percent of the tumor. In the distance is another step – Gamma Knife radiation to achieve further reduction.

After four weeks of rehabilitation at the medical center, Toni returns home to continue it. Loss of hearing in the right ear, further disturbance to the right eye, having to be fed through a tube in her stomach because of throat damage, and weakness that affects her balance in walking are among the tough negatives with which she has to deal.

Her recovery progress over ensuing months is so remarkable that she is ready for Gamma Knife treatment at the University of Virginia Health Science Center in Charlottesville. This takes place in the fall of 1994. Follow-up MRIs show further reductions in the tumor.

What comes through from Toni's incredible medical journey is how three forces have combined to produce the miracle that she is alive and living a normal life:

- the extraordinary skills of modern medical science;
- her own positive, upbeat courage, determination, and faith;
- the understanding, support, and strength she consistently received from family and friends.

What she unfolds regarding these forces holds great benefit not only for other patients, but for those close to them.

1

The Beginning

"Toni, I've noticed how often you move your head up and down and rub the back of your neck. Tell me – is something wrong?"

It should have come as no surprise that my friend Jeanie would ask this question. We'd been together many times during the early part of 1991. And it was in January that I first felt a strange sensation in the back of my neck. It wasn't painful – just sort of a dull ache, more annoying than disturbing. It would come and go. Moving my head up and down and rubbing my neck had become an automatic response to it.

"No, Jeanie," I assured her. "Everything is all right. It's just a funny ache I get in the back of my neck. It's probably a reaction to stress – trying to get so many things done every day. I haven't caught up since Christmas."

Jeanie obviously wasn't fully satisfied with my explanation. But she didn't pursue the matter. And I certainly didn't have the slightest premonition that my recurring neck ache was an indication of the incredible experiences lying ahead of me over the next four years.

As anyone with a household of four children knows, stress is a part of everyday life for a mother. At the time, our four ranged in age from 7 to 17. Wonderful, busy children I love deeply, they did keep me endlessly in motion – driving, delivering, shopping, supervising, reminding, feeding, and all the rest. Often I would fall into bed at night utterly exhausted, but always grateful that we had been blessed with this family.

Adding to the stress factor, I was a "weekday widow." In his work, my husband Richard had to do a great deal of traveling. So I also had the responsibility of being head of the household much of the time. In addition, I had my own PTA activities and served once a week as an after-school teacher with the Confraternity of Christian Doctrine at my church.

So, with all that was going on every day, it seemed logical to assume my neck aches were a reflection of built-up stress from trying to do too many things in too few hours. How wrong this self-diagnosis turned out to be! If only the whole thing had been that simple.

Another Signal

With no let-up in the recurrence of this ache as the winter weeks went by, I began thinking about a rear-end car collision I had been in a few months before. Had there been some whiplash from it? Rather than stress, could my neck problem be a delayed reaction from the accident? I decided to find out and made an appointment with a chiropractor.

He agreed that it could be a result of whiplash and set to work on my spine. All told, I went to him about a dozen times, with appointments two or three days each week. The ache would go away for a while, but would always come back a short time later. Yet, X-rays he took of my spine showed no visible problem.

In the spring something rather disturbing began happening. Sometimes when I would get out of my car I would have a strange feeling of disorientation. My balance wasn't affected, but for about 30 seconds I seemed to be floating. It was as if I were in space instead of standing on the ground. Then suddenly I was back. Never, never had I experienced anything so eerie. While this didn't occur every time I got out of the car, it did happen on enough occasions to tell me something was wrong.

What could it be? I had no pains anywhere. I felt healthy. I would get tired, yes. But that was nothing new. I was sure any woman would get tired from my daily schedule. What on earth could be wrong?

By coincidence, Richard had asked me to go with him in May to a convention at the Greenbrier Hotel in White Sulphur Springs, West Virginia. The Greenbrier has a medical clinic for health checkups. We decided to leave three days early so both of us could take advantage of it and find out what I wanted and needed to know.

The doctors there gave us clean bills of health, but were perplexed about my strange sensations. They suggested that after we returned home, I go for an MRI to get a picture of what might be going on inside my brain. It wasn't an urgent enough recommendation to cause any alarm, so we didn't let it dampen our enjoyment of being at that lovely resort in the mountains of West Virginia.

Forced Action

Although I knew it would be wise to have an MRI and actually find out what might be wrong, I put off doing anything about it. As usual, there were so many other things to do, and as I look back, perhaps I really didn't want to know what was going on. But soon I was given no choice in the matter.

Our 17-year-old son Lee had broken his ankle roller blading. He was being treated by Dr. Steve O'Brien, an orthopedic surgeon and family friend in Garden City. In June, I took Lee to him for a check of the healing ankle. While there, I decided to tell Steve about the neck aches and the strange episodes of disorientation.

He asked me questions about them – how long they had been occurring, how often, how I felt otherwise. Obviously, from the serious tone of his voice, he was concerned about them. His firmness left no doubt that I should be doing something.

"You're going to a neurologist. What's more, I'm going to make the appointment for you right now."

I was surprised at this. "Do you think there could be something serious?"

He remained firm. "I don't know, but we're going to find out. The fact you've had these symptoms for some months tells me it's time to see what they mean. And the only way to do that is to get to a specialist who can tell."

He excused himself, went into another room, and in a few minutes was back.

"All right, you're set. I've made an appointment for you with Dr. Peter Tsaris in New York. I've told him what you've explained to me, and he does want to see you. He's thorough. He'll tell you what you should know if he finds something. Believe me, it's the only smart thing to do."

All along, the children had known about the neck aches, but I always had passed them off lightly as being nothing serious. I hadn't told them, though, about the disorientation episodes. Now Lee knew I had symptoms serious enough to call for a trip to a neurologist for examination. He was upset about it, but on the way home, we agreed not to say anything to the other children. There would be time for that after I had been to New York.

I have often thought back to that day in Steve O'Brien's office. It was his insistence that started me on a medical odyssey I couldn't possibly have imagined having to travel. Difficult and traumatic as the journey has been, I am so thankful to him for getting me underway. If he hadn't, I might have been on a trip into darkness.

A Visible Clue

Richard was away, and Jeanie volunteered to go with me to New York for my appointment with Dr. Tsaris. I was delighted to have her. We decided to drive the 25 miles from Garden City.

On the way in, we avoided talking about the appointment. Both of us knew it was best to keep my mind on other things. So we discussed our families, our plans for the summer, the newest fashions, anything but the reason for this trip.

Once in the doctor's office, though, I faced the day's reality. I was there to find out about my mysterious symptoms. At this point I really wanted to know so I could get on with whatever needed to be done about them.

How very much skilled medical practitioners deserve our admiration. Dr. Tsaris examined my head and my neck with the utmost care and precision. Then he turned to my eyes with the test of following his finger as he moved it to different angles from my face. It was there that he detected the only clue visible to him. It was a slight fluttering movement in my right eye. This led him to suspect something might be occurring inside my brain.

How calm he was about it and how very much I appreciated his calmness. "Let's find out what's going on. I'll arrange for an immediate MRI. It's best to get it now while you're in the city."

For the first time, I couldn't hold back a feeling of anxiety. "What could be going on inside my head?"

He still was calm, expressing no concern. "We can't know until we look. The MRI will tell us."

It took little time for arrangements to be made for the MRI. Dr. Tsaris gave me the address, only a block from his office; Jeanie and I were there in just a few minutes.

Window on the Brain

What is it like to have an MRI? I've been asked this question many times. The best answer I've found is to tell about my first experience.

After we arrived for my scheduled appointment that day, one of the technicians briefed me on "magnetic resonance imaging," MRI for short, an amazing product of modern technology and medical science. I learned, though I don't have much of a scientific mind, how it performs the miracle of revealing details about the body's inner structures and organs.

Inside a large cylinder in which I would be lying, electric magnets would expose the tissues in my brain to short bursts from a combination of powerful, but not harmful, magnetic fields and radio waves. These bursts would stimulate the tissues to send signals which would be analyzed by computer and con-verted to remarkably clear pictures. Examining these pictures would reveal anything that could explain the symptoms I had been having and the unusual eye fluttering Dr. Tsaris had detected.

In one of several small rooms with lockers, I undressed, and put on a hospital gown. No jewelry could be worn nor anything else with metal on it.

Inside the room with the big MRI cylinder, I got up onto a long, table-like platform at the entry end of the cylinder and lay on my back. Technicians in attendance put a support under my knees to relieve back pressure. Then I was given a set of head phones and a long-corded panic button to keep in my hand. Next, a blanket was put over me for use if I felt cold.

I was told the procedure would take 30 minutes. My head would have to be perfectly still all the time. I could move my feet and cross my ankles, however, to help ease any tension I might feel from being so motionless.

The technicians said they would talk to me through the head phones and explain things along the way; also they could hear me if I wanted to talk to them. It was then that they put a sort of cage over my head. It had a mirror inside so I would be able to see myself. If I pressed the panic button, I could be out of the machine in seconds.

Hydraulic action moved the platform with me on it into the cylinder to a point needed for the first set of pictures. It was explained through the head phones that there would be a series of pictures taken. Each picture would take between two and six minutes. In all cases, I would be told just what the length would be.

Each picture began with four loud clicks, signals that the imaging was starting. These were followed by rapid clicks for as long as the specific view required. I quickly found out how noisy the MRI mechanism can be and followed advice the technicians had given me about keeping the head phones on and listening to music.

When the first series was completed, I was told the table I was lying on would be moved slightly toward the cylinder's opening. This repositioning, which occurred twice, was to focus the magnetic action on different areas of my brain in order to get the most relevant pictures.

Music came through the head phones between explanations, and a happy coincidence made it especially absorbing and relaxing for me. There were songs that our son Lee, who played guitar and keyboard, would often sing. One, "Browneyed Girl," always made me think of our then 12-year-old daughter Susan. The other was "Wonderful Tonight." I was so surprised to hear those two very special songs inside that cylinder. It was almost as if they had been planned.

After the first 15 minutes, I was moved entirely out of the cylinder for a substance called gadolinium to be injected into my arm. I was told this was a form of dye, or contrast agent, that travels through the arteries and veins. In the brain, it highlights and verifies abnormal vessel formations which occur commonly with tumors. Then back into the cylinder I went for another 15 minutes of the same procedure as before.

The whole thing was really not an ordeal. There was no pain. And I was sure the pictures wouldn't show anything serious that couldn't be taken care of with medication.

Until the images had been "read" thoroughly, I wouldn't know the actual results. The pictures and an analysis of them would be sent to Dr. Tsaris. He would call and let me know what they showed. Meanwhile, the glorious days of summer were here and it was Thursday. Jeanie and I were thinking and talking about the coming weekend as we drove back, not about MRI results.

The Shock

Friday was the last day of school. The children would be out early, but each had plans and wouldn't be home until evening. I was busy all morning running errands and getting ready for the weekend. My mood was happy and far away from neck aches and disorientations.

Richard had come home early from his trip and was outside when the telephone rang in mid-afternoon. I answered it with no thought Dr. Tsaris would be on the line; I had assumed there wouldn't be word from him until sometime the following week. But it was his voice I heard. And the shock from what he told me will remain forever embedded in my memory.

"I have bad and good news for you. The bad news is that a large tumor has grown at the base of your brain. The good news is that it very likely is benign."

The words stunned me so that I went blank. I don't know what I said to him. He went on to ask me to call him the next week about an appointment with a neurosurgeon. The tumor would have to be removed. It would require major surgery.

Normally, I could keep my emotions pretty well under control. Not this time. I had so convinced myself there could be nothing seriously wrong that I wasn't up to the sudden news this had been a false hope. In little more than a minute, the brightness of a day filled with thoughts of a happy summer weekend had clouded into darkness. How long I sat by the telephone crying, I don't know. When Richard came back in, he found me there.

It was so hard to tell him what I had heard on that telephone, so difficult to say the frightening words – *brain tumor*. But he had to know.

His reaction was shocked disbelief. "Tumor? Toni, Toni, it can't be! How can it be?"

Richard rushed over and took me in his arms. The comfort of having him close helped tremendously. But I couldn't stop crying. If I had thought there could be even a remote possibility that I might have a tumor on my brain, it would have been my worst fear. We stayed there for a few minutes, and I was still sobbing when Lee walked into the room. His plans had changed and he was home earlier than expected. I remember the sudden surprise on his face when he looked at me – and his quick, anxious questions. It was the first time he had ever seen me cry.

"Mom, you're crying. What's wrong? What's happened?"

Since he had been with me when Steve O'Brien had made my appointment with Dr. Tsaris, we knew we must tell him about the telephone call. More calmly than I would have been able to do it, Richard explained about the MRI and what it had found.

Lee's reaction was the same as ours had been. It was such a shock. It never had entered our minds there could be anything like this. I did manage to stop sobbing, though, and the three of us talked about what we should say to the other children – Michael, two years younger than Lee, Susan, and Richard II, 7. We decided there was no need to upset them at this point. It would be better to wait until we ourselves knew more.

A short time later, I called my younger sister Maryann who, with her husband Dan, lives nearby. She had made me promise to let her know the MRI results as soon as I had word on them.

Again, I couldn't hold back the tears when I told her about the call from Dr. Tsaris. But she was so loving and genuine in the support and encouragement she gave me that I received a real lift from talking with her. This was only the first of countless things Maryann and Dan have done, not only for me but for the entire family, to help us throughout my long medical journey.

After our talk, I sat by the telephone thinking about my situation. I just couldn't get over the devastating blow of hearing that I had a brain tumor. I was scared, terribly scared. Major surgery? Obviously, I not only had a tumor, but it had to be a critically serious one to require major surgery! I tried to keep negative thoughts from my mind, but I couldn't. Would there be a question of surviving? Or, perhaps even worse, might my brain be permanently damaged?

It was undoubtedly a natural reaction to be consumed with such fears. But as they intensified, I began to realize that I was doing exactly the wrong thing. I was assuming the worst without having any basis for doing so. It was then that I told myself that I had to be rational, ask questions, get the facts, and proceed from there.

Reflections

Make Sure of the Diagnosis

The first need is the extremely important one of securing an accurate diagnosis. Because of the pressure they can build up in the brain, especially the compression of areas next to them, all brain tumors are serious. Only by actually seeing the growth itself and its precise location can there be the right decision on how best to perform surgery or use radiation on it.

Don't be afraid of the MRI machine if that is the method of imaging required to reveal necessary details about your condition. Everything is done by the attending staff to help the patient stay calm and comfortable, and there are aids for persons with claustrophobia.

You Are Not Alone

It isn't a simple matter to suppress anxiety and fear upon learning the startling fact that a tumor has grown inside your brain. But it is a good thing to avoid any inclination to feel sorry for yourself as having been "singled out."

At the time of my diagnosis, I hadn't the faintest idea how prevalent brain surgery was. Later, I read that every year in this country more than 100,000 people are diagnosed with brain tumors. And there are close to a million cases of brain-related surgery annually. So, it *is* important to keep in mind that many others have gone through – and survived in good health – what you are facing.

2

Reality And Decision

No Sad Songs

Before the other children arrived home that Friday afternoon, I also called Jeanie. As I picked up the telephone, I thought back to the time months before when she had asked me whether something was wrong. I knew she hadn't been satisfied with my explanation that the ache in the back of my neck probably was nothing more than a reaction to stress. But that was what I had been naive enough to think.

Even though she had suspected something more than that, it was a blow to her to hear about the brain tumor. True to her loyal nature, she said she would drop everything to be there whenever I needed her. As a free-lance interior designer, her hours were flexible. It was comforting to know I always could count on her to help. How little we anticipated then how much her help would mean to all of us for such a long time.

The next morning, after all the children were out of the house, Richard and I told our wonderful Elena.

Years before, shortly after her arrival from El Salvador, she had come to work for us. She could speak little English then, but was so willing to learn and so helpful in so many ways that she became a treasured part of our family.

She was pained by the news we gave her about the tumor, but strong as she hugged me tightly. "Oh, Mrs. Ferrucci, I will take care of you and the children. Don't you worry. You will be all right. I will pray hard for you."

We explained to her that Lee knew about the tumor, but we were going to wait to tell Susan, Michael, and Richard II until after I had been to New York for another medical appointment. She understood why we wanted to wait, and we knew we could trust her to say nothing until after we had talked with them.

Then we turned to something else. A dinner party had been planned at our house for Saturday evening of the coming Fourth of July weekend. It was to be for our friend Joe Ingarra's wife Colleen who was soon to have a baby. Should the dinner be cancelled? It did seem illogical for someone who just had learned she had a serious brain tumor to be staging a party a few days later.

On the other hand, why not go ahead with it? I had made up my mind to be rational about the tumor, and not jump to conclusions until I had the facts. There certainly was no need to go into seclusion.

This decision, unimportant as it might seem, was actually a great plus. I knew there was no way I could blot out the news that a threatening object had grown inside my brain. But I couldn't let fear possess my every thought and action. That would only lead to feeling sorry for myself – something I knew I must avoid.

A New Experience

Two friends, Carolyn Casano and Nora Forrelli, were helping with the party. Carolyn's son Chris and Nora's son Richard were Lee's best friends. Though it turned out he didn't, I was concerned that Lee might confide in the boys about the tumor. Just in case this happened, I thought I'd better let their mothers know. A convenient opportunity presented itself on Monday when the three of us got together to go over some of our plans for Saturday evening.

Both were shaken by the news, and they had all kinds of anxious questions. What had caused the tumor? How did it feel? How long would I be in the hospital? What could they do to help? What about the children? These were questions I couldn't answer until I knew more. As for the party, they were sure I wouldn't want to go through with it.

My answer was definite. "Oh yes, I do. I want to go on with everything we've planned. I've made up my mind not to let worry about the tumor take control of my life. I'm going to keep just as busy as I can."

They were surprised that I was so determined about it. But they went along with me in my wish that we should act as if nothing had changed.

Staying busy was easy. With summer vacation under way, the children had lots of activities and I did plenty of driving to get them places and pick them up later. Maryann came over several times and we had lunch or went shopping. Jeanie had an interesting new decorating assignment, and we spent time together while she looked for fabrics. And, of course, there always was grocery shopping to do, to say nothing of cooking. By no means was the tumor entirely out of my thoughts. But I did manage to hold to my positive perspective. I actively tried to keep myself absorbed and busy with both everyday chores and special plans.

The Saturday-evening party was a new test. Could I spend the whole evening acting as if nothing at all had happened? By then, everyone there knew about the tumor. Some seemed surprised that I hadn't changed in appearance or mental state. It probably was natural to think I somehow would be different from the last time they had seen me. I suspect they wondered how I really felt inside. Regardless of this, everyone cooperated in not saying or doing anything to dampen the festivity of an evening filled with happiness for Colleen and Joe. This helped me to pass the test.

Every time I have seen the handsome little boy who was born a short time later, I have thought of that evening. It was a prelude to embarking on a procession of experiences that I couldn't possibly have envisioned at the time.

The Pictures

Meanwhile, Dr. Tsaris had made an appointment for me with Dr. Michael Lavyne, a neurosurgeon at New York Hospital. It was set for Wednesday, July 10th.

Richard went with me. I must admit that some pangs of apprehension did flash across my mind as we drove into the city. Now that we were to get more information on the tumor, what would the reality be? We would soon know.

Dr. Lavyne, personable and friendly, took us into his office shortly after we arrived. There wasn't the slightest hint of gloom in the warm way he approached what he had to tell us, and this was encouraging.

First, he showed us the MRI pictures. We saw a side view of my head inside the skull, almost as if the flesh and skull on the entire side of my face had been removed. Also, there were skeleton-like pictures of the same type looking in from the top of my head down into the brain. An unskilled eye would not have picked up any abnormality, but Dr. Lavyne pointed to a mass area that stood out because it was darker. It was the tumor. We were amazed at how large it was, about the size of a lemon. It was at the base of my brain leading down into the spinal cord, filling in what should have been an empty space.

Dr. Lavyne explained that there are different types of brain tumors and the characteristics of each tell the surgeon what has to be done to remove it. Mine was called a meningioma. As we learned later, this meant it had arisen from cells in the middle layer of the meninges, the three membranes covering and protecting the brain and the spinal cord. He went on to say this type of tumor, found most commonly in adult women, was slow-growing, different from more aggressive ones that arise from the brain's substance.

We were astonished when he told us I probably had had the tumor for many years, possibly even had been born with it. It was incredible that an object had grown to such a size inside my head without my being aware of it.

He also pointed out that the brain is a structure in a fixed space, the skull, and it can tolerate only so much added volume from a tumor. Mine had reached the pressure stage, accounting for the recurring neck ache and the episodes of disorientation that made me feel as if I were floating in space. These not only were symptoms, but warning signs. At some point, buildup of more pressure would swell the brain further and perhaps even pierce the skull.

There was definitely no option. I would have to have an operation. And because of the tumor's location, highly delicate surgery would be required. Extreme care would have to be taken to avoid disturbing the brainstem's vital network of nerves that serve as the communication system between the brain and the rest of the body. Moreover, avoiding such disturbance would mean some of the tumor would have to be left.

Although there was no question about my having to undergo an operation, Dr. Lavyne said it wouldn't have to be done right away. The tumor was not life-threatening. We could take some time to think about it and make plans. He pointed out that he himself concentrated on back surgery, and therefore would not attempt the type of operation I required. When we were leaving, he said something that seemed both advice and a caution: "Don't let anyone tell you the whole tumor can be removed."

We were taken aback by what we had learned, but appreciated the calm, frank way Dr. Lavyne had explained things to us. There would be much to think and talk about later under better circumstances. Late-afternoon Long Island traffic wasn't conducive to anything except concentrating on getting from New York to Garden City safely.

One thing we did decide before we finally arrived home was to let Lee and Elena know what we had found out, but to delay talking with the other three children. The better time for that, we thought, would be after we knew when and where I would be having the operation.

So, acting as if nothing out of the ordinary had happened during the day, we had a normal, though later-than-usual, family dinner. As we were to discover along the way, however, it was a mistake not to have been entirely open with Susan, Michael, and Richard II from the very beginning. We were to learn a lesson that

will be of value for *all* patients who have young
children.

Night Images

After everyone else had gone to bed, Richard and I
went into the kitchen and closed the door. We could talk
there without being overheard in any other part of the
house. Richard asked me how I felt about what Dr.
Lavyne had told us now that a few hours had passed.

My thoughts were actually somewhat mixed.
Naturally I was upset about an operation that would
obviously be long and difficult. But as I thought about
what we had seen in the MRI pictures and the calm way
Dr. Lavyne had explained about the tumor, I didn't
have the same feeling of fear that had gripped me
when I first learned about it. Difficult surgery? Others
had faced it and survived. So could I. The right thing to
do, and what I made up my mind to do, was to take a
positive attitude toward the surgery and resolve to go
ahead with faith and confidence in the outcome.

There was no way of knowing then how many
times this attitude would be tested by some steep hills
and sharp curves in the long journey. But through the
ups and downs, I have made myself resolutely cling to
it. This has been my key to survival. And how fortunate
I have been that it has radiated to the many others
whose understanding and support have been of invaluable help along the way.

What did concern me was that the operation could
mean a long hospital stay. How would the household

manage without me? I had always been a take-charge person. With the children, I had been at the emergency room when there was an injury, up all night when they were sick, by their sides to help with school work, ready and willing in so many other ways.

How would all these things be done if I had to be away from home for some time? I knew Elena would take good care of the children and do everything else she possibly could. But she didn't drive a car, and there was so much driving involved in our daily lives. I couldn't expect Maryann and my friends to take on these and other responsibilities, much as I knew they would cut into their own busy schedules to help.

Richard assured me everything could be worked out and not to worry about it. He said – and he was right – the most important thing we had to do now was find the right neurosurgeon to do the operation. Since we didn't have to rush into it, he would begin making some calls to get names.

It was probably inevitable that sleep wouldn't come easily that night. I lay awake for some time after we went to bed. The MRI images we had seen in Dr. Lavyne's office kept flickering across my mind as if they were on a television screen. The tumor was more prominent than it had been in the actual pictures. And, as the images repeated themselves, it gradually grew in size, dominating them more and more. I tried to concentrate on other things, but there was no turnoff button I could press. I couldn't let this go on. But what could I do to stop it?

The screen-like flickering gave me an idea. I never had been one to watch late-night television. Usually I was too tired at the end of the day to think about anything other than sleep. On this night that changed. I got up, went downstairs, and turned the television on.

It was a surprise to find such an assortment of things to watch. I settled on a movie from the 1950s, "Roman Holiday," starring Audrey Hepburn and Gregory Peck. It was a delightful film, and I became so totally absorbed in it that there was no room for other images. I watched to the very end. Back upstairs in bed I still had happy movie scenes in my mind. I had found an escape. This was to be one of many nights when I was grateful to makers of happy movies of the past. Quite a change from years before when I was up with a new baby and there was nothing but snow on TV!

An Incident

The next morning, I knew I had to spend some time making telephone calls. I had promised to let Maryann, Jeanie, and others know what we had learned from Dr. Lavyne. When all the children were out of the house I sat down at the kitchen table to begin. Just as I was picking up the telephone, I heard a car in the driveway and saw that it was Carolyn Casano and her daughter Carrie.

Carolyn was one of the friends I had been going to call, and I was so glad to see her there that I went right out to greet her. Her voice was anxious. "Toni, what did you find out yesterday? I almost called you last night, but thought maybe I shouldn't."

"We learned that it's a very large tumor and we have to see about an operation." I was pleased with my calm answer.

"How large?"

"It's about the size of a lemon."

"A lemon? Oh, my God!"

Suddenly she stiffened. A panicky look came over her face. In an instant she was out of the car. Breathing heavily, she paced up and down as if to stabilize herself. I knew she suffered from severe claustrophobia. Hearing about the size of the tumor and thinking about an operation to get it out had apparently overcome her. But in a few minutes she was all right.

She put her arms around me. There was a choke in her voice when she spoke. "You know Charlie and I will do anything to help. Anything. Will you please let us know? When do you expect to find out about the operation?"

"We really don't know. We have to find a surgeon. Richard is going to make some calls and we'll have to see what develops. We do have some time. It doesn't have to be done right away."

Many times since, we've joked about her reaction in the driveway. But there were no laughs then.

After they left, I did get to the phone to call Maryann, Jeanie, and Nora. All were startled when I told them about the size of the tumor. But, for the most part, the conversations were calm. Like Carolyn, everyone wanted to know how and when they could help, assuring me they would come anywhere, any time I needed them. There were some tears, not from talking about the tumor, but from my being so deeply touched by knowing how genuine they were and how blessed I was to have them.

A Coincidence

When Richard and I were alone later that evening, he told me about several calls he had made during the day to get leads on surgeons. He would continue his search until he had to be away part of the following week.

On Sunday, Richard and the boys went to an early-morning ball game. They would go to church later. Meanwhile, Susan and I went to the early service. As we were leaving the church, I was surprised to see my friend Anne Keating across the way. She noticed me at the same time, and we made our way through the crowd to greet each other.

Anne and I had been in school together and always had kept in contact. She lived in New York and all of us were proud of her successful business career. She had risen to become vice president of one of the city's most famous stores. She said she was spending the weekend at her parents' home on Long Island and had been planning to call me that afternoon.

It was fate to have run into each other this way. Anne and I always had much to talk about. When she asked how our summer was going, I couldn't hold back the tears even before I told her about the tumor. She was as shocked as the rest of us had been.

"Toni, you? A brain tumor? I can't believe it. You look so healthy. Is there anything I can do?"

"I really don't know. Richard is checking on neurosurgeons. We want to find the right one."

"Let me check something for you. Joan Kearny, a girl I know in Westchester County, had a brain tumor and loved the doctor who operated on her. I don't know his name, but I'll find out. Joan said he's one of the very best neurosurgeons."

This was good to hear and I asked her to please get his name. I was so encouraged that I could hardly wait to tell Richard. I knew Anne would follow through.

She called me that very afternoon. The surgeon was Dr. Richard Fraser, of New York Hospital. Again she said how pleased her friend Joan was with what he had done for her. She gave me Joan's telephone number and suggested I call her.

That day I did call Joan Kearny. She was very enthusiastic in her comments about Dr. Fraser. Her tumor had not been the same as mine, but it had been a hard one to remove. She said she had been scared before the operation, but it had been a great success. She was glad I had called and told me to try not to worry. I was heartened by having talked with someone who actually had been through the experience and had come out of it so well.

Through contacts in New York, Richard found that Dr. Fraser indeed was regarded as a leading neurosurgeon, not only in New York, but nationally. We agreed that Richard should try to make an appointment with him. With a man as busy as Dr. Fraser, this didn't turn out to be easy, but Richard succeeded in making an appointment for late July.

We arrived at his office on the set day, and when he shook our hands, both of us were immediately impressed with this fine doctor. His easily approachable, warm manner made us feel confident about the interview.

After we talked a few minutes about my MRI pictures which he had in front of him, he took me into an adjoining examination room. As I sat on a table, he tested my arm, elbow, and knee reflexes. He also had me do the finger-to-nose test, as well as the eye maneuver of watching his moving finger. Then he had me walk so he could observe my balance.

When we sat down again in his office, he emphasized that in his opinion this tumor had reached a stage where it had to come out. Precision would be required in such a delicate operation. I'll never forget his words;

"There's no making mistakes in brain surgery."

He said he always told his students that a foot of the intestine could be removed without causing trouble. But not a half inch of the brain.

Then we received some sobering news. He said he was obligated to tell us that there would be risks in an operation as complex as mine would be. He wanted us to be fully aware of them. I possibly could lose the sight in one eye. One ear could be deaf. And there was a possibility of facial paralysis.

These were not only unhappy, but surprising things to hear. Even after we had learned from Dr. Lavyne about the critical location of the tumor, I naively had assumed everything would be perfectly normal after an operation to remove it. Now, hearing this could be far from true, I was getting my first lesson in the importance of knowing and understanding the medical side of the picture – what was involved and *why*.

At that moment in the doctor's office, the one thing I could cling to was his saying there *could* be these effects. They weren't certainties. And the reality was that I had no choice anyway. The tumor couldn't be left in my brain just because I didn't want to face the risks entailed in removing it.

The only question left to be answered was whether Dr. Fraser would perform the operation. There was no doubt in our minds about wanting him to be the surgeon to do it, and we were relieved when he said he would.

Now it was only a matter of setting a date. Our son Lee had enrolled as a freshman at the University of Colorado in Boulder and would be going there late in August. I had been hoping to go with him to help him get settled for his new life as a college student, so I asked Dr. Fraser whether the operation could be put off until September. He said this would be no problem, and checking his schedule, set Thursday, September 12th as the date.

In preparation for the operation, I was to start two weeks before on steroids to prevent swelling in my brain during the surgery. He gave me a prescription, and I was to take three pills a day during the two-week period.

Two big steps had been taken. We had our surgeon and we had a date. The third would be the operation itself.

Reflections

Get the Details

A lesson many patients have learned is the importance of asking questions – all kinds of pertinent questions – beginning with the first examination by a doctor. The more information found out about the case, the better prepared and equipped you are to deal with the surgery itself and with possible aftereffects. Getting as much information as possible about the type and location of the tumor is especially important. This knowledge helps you to understand why certain things have to be done and why they might cause adverse effects.

I have often heard people say they don't ask their doctor for more details because there isn't time. It certainly is true that many medical professionals are extraordinarily busy. But in my experience and from what I have read, there seems to be a trend to do more to meet the patients' need for information. In my case, I didn't know things I should have from the beginning because I didn't ask enough questions.

3

A Time for Learning

Needed Perspective

Richard and I were silent as we drove home that afternoon in the heavy Long Island commuter traffic. There was much to think about. The more we were learning about the tumor, the more there was to consider about the operation. For one thing, the negatives Dr. Fraser mentioned were beginning to take hold of me.

The loss of sight in one eye. What would this mean? Would I be totally blind in that eye or would I have partial sight? How would it look? Would other people be able to tell? How about driving? I've always spent so much time in the car. We take so many things for granted until we have to think of what it would be like to get along without them.

Certainly I wouldn't want to lose any sight at all, but if that were the price I had to pay to be free of the tumor, I'd live with that.

Loss of hearing in one ear. Again, this was something hard to imagine, simply because there'd never been any need to think about it. Now, it might have to be faced. As with my eye, it would have to be considered a matter of giving up a precious possession to be rid of the tumor. I would have to learn to compensate.

Facial paralysis. This was scary. Would my face be contorted? Would I look freakish? Would I be ashamed to let people see me? All sorts of nightmarish thoughts quickly were triggered by the ominous prospect of a face frozen in position.

I had to keep reminding myself that these were only possibilities, things that *could* happen, not definitely etched in stone. There was no certainty about facial paralysis, loss of sight in one eye, loss of hearing in one ear. I had to hope and believe they wouldn't occur, but be ready to confront them with a positive attitude and try to deal successfully with them if they did happen.

Inside the Family

Now that the operation was set, we knew we couldn't put off any longer telling Susan and Michael about the tumor. Lee, of course, already knew. With Richard II, we thought we could wait until just before I would be going to the hospital and ask the others not to mention it to him until we had talked with him.

We weren't sure of how far we should go in telling Susan and Michael. We wondered how important it was for them to know how serious the operation would be. And should they be warned about the possible things Dr. Fraser had told us could occur? Thinking about such injuries to their mother would upset them for the rest of the summer. Was it fair to do that to them? On the other hand, would it be fair not to tell them the full story? As members of our close family, weren't they entitled to know?

We were in a dilemma and not sure of the right way out of it. The best course seemed to be to say I had gone for tests to find the cause of my neck pains and a tumor had been found. I would have to have an operation in September to remove it. We wouldn't say anything about the possible aftereffects. We would hope there wouldn't be any and that it would have been unnecessary and wrong to upset them.

Richard felt he should talk with them alone. He probably sensed that emotion might take over if I tried to tell them and would create exactly the kind of reaction we didn't want. Since I wasn't entirely sure how well I could handle the situation, I willingly agreed to his doing it on his own.

An opportunity occurred that evening after I had gone upstairs with Richard II to help get him ready for a camping trip he was taking the next morning. When I returned alone a little while later, Susan and Michael came to me together. Both kissed me and said how sorry they were I would have to have an operation, but were glad it would stop my neck aches. I was happy to see they weren't unduly upset. Richard had carried out his mission well.

Susan kept looking at the back of my neck. "Did the doctor say the operation would leave a scar on your neck?" she asked. "If it does, I hope it will just be a small one."

What could I say to that? She said it for me. I loved her for her sensitivity in not wanting her mother to have a scar showing.

They wanted to know how long I would be in the hospital. All I could say was I didn't know, but hoped it wouldn't be for long. Both told me not to worry about them while I was away. Everything would be all right. They and Elena would take care of things. And could they come to see me right after the operation? They would want to be there. Understandable questions but unanswerable at this point.

As we were to discover later, it was a mistake not to have been entirely open and frank with them about everything from the beginning. They deserved our confidence in being able to cope with the full truth. We should have shown that confidence in them.

Our mothers also were to be considered. Up to this time we had said nothing to either of them, Richard's in Connecticut, mine in Florida, both widows.

We knew Richard's mother, Jo, would be extremely emotional about it. Perhaps we should keep the whole thing from her until after the operation. The more we talked about it, the more this seemed the best for her. But it wasn't. She was upset and wished we had told her. She felt she could have helped.

As for my mother Estelle, I decided to telephone Chris, a close friend of hers in Florida and ask his advice. I knew she would insist on being with us at the time of the operation. But the question was how far in advance to tell her, knowing how much it would worry and upset her.

Her friend had a good solution. He said he had to come north early in September. He would suggest to her that she fly with him to New York. He had work to do there and she could be on Long Island visiting us and Maryann and Dan. This would give us an opportunity to tell her the story face to face before the operation, much better than my explaining it to her on the telephone. Meanwhile, he would keep it to himself. With Mom happy to come to Long Island for a visit, this was the plan we followed.

Wanting to Know

Although the operation was some weeks away, I began thinking of plans and preparations that would have to be made for taking care of things at home while I was at the hospital in New York. So, I started what turned out to be an ongoing "To Do" list. At the same time, there was a sort of nagging desire – or perhaps need – that made me long for a real understanding of the brain itself and of the tumor that had intruded on mine.

The MRI images Dr. Lavyne had shown us and the explanations he and Dr. Fraser had given us had been clear for the moment. We had listened, but had asked absolutely no questions. Our minds were so absorbed with the realization I had a tumor to be removed that we couldn't think about anything else. But time had changed this, and now I was thinking more deeply about the situation. I wanted a full visualization of the brain's inner structure and the exact location of the tumor.

This was the first curiosity of such depth that I had felt. Up to this point, the need had been to get the problem identified and find out how it could be handled. Now that we knew both answers, I wanted to get myself better informed on just what was going to be taking place inside my brain. In short, a desire for medical information had arisen and I made up my mind to satisfy it. As I look back, I'm glad the curiosity developed. It is surprising how valuable simple medical information can be in helping to keep a positive attitude.

She hadn't said anything about it before, but I soon learned from Maryann that she had already done some exploring.

"I went over to the library yesterday to see what type of information is available on the brain, tumor operations, and anything else that's important," she said. "The more we know about the medical side of the whole thing, the better equipped we'll be in handling whatever we have to face."

We were on the same track. "I couldn't agree with you more. Were you able to find material that you could understand?"

Her answer was enthusiastic. "They have a terrific medical encyclopedia that's wonderfully illustrated. The explanations are clear and extremely helpful in answering obvious questions. I made some notes. Maybe you will want to do the same thing. Then we can get together and compare our findings."

This was the right approach for me, and I decided to go the next day to tackle the medical encyclopedia. In fact, I found myself really looking forward to it. I knew I wouldn't get much sleep that night thinking about the knowledge I was soon to gain.

Inside Views

The lesson I gave myself in the library the next day was even more satisfying than the expectation I had built for it. The medical encyclopedia, published by the American Medical Association, was just where Maryann had told me I would find it. With almost 1200 pages, there was an impressive amount of information between its covers.

As I opened the pages to the section on the brain, my reaction with what I saw first was fascination. There were remarkably vivid sketches of the interior of the wondrous organ. By using color effectively, they detailed with marked clarity the location, shape, and size of each separate area or region. Accompanying them were clear, precise descriptions of the function of each.

Also there were photos showing examples of interior views obtained by three common methods of imaging: MRI, angiography, and CT scan, the latter two using X-ray photography. For any patient or student, these pictures demonstrated the values of the different methods of looking inside. Truly a picture is worth a thousand words!

After studying the sketches for several minutes and making a number of notes from them, I began reading the full text. As I moved along, I became more and more aware of how little I knew about the magnificent organ responsible for our thought, speech, and emotions, along with serving as the body's control center.

There was a faint recollection of having learned at least a little about all this at some point in school. Unfortunately, though, with so much to assimilate along the way, the tendency is to take mental and physical processes for granted and seldom think about them until something happens. There was no question about this having been the case with me.

The text included descriptions of different kinds of brain tumors. Just as had been explained to us, I read that mine was called a meningioma. This was because it had arisen from one of the brain-covering meningeal membranes. This type, nearly always benign, can be multiple in number and can be at different locations in the brain. At other locations, these tumors logically can be dealt with more easily than when they are on the brainstem.

From what I read, I knew that since the tumor had grown to such a size, it made something unmistakably clear – it had to come out. Located in such a vulnerable position on the brainstem, the pressure it could exert in different ways would be dangerous to the brain itself and to my entire body. This location emphasized how difficult and delicate the operation would be.

One could not have a lesson of this kind without being impressed by the functioning of the brain and central nervous system. When Maryann and I compared our notes, we had the understanding we both needed for my case. With it, I felt much better equipped mentally for the coming operation.

In fact, I felt so much more comfortable from having done some research that I wondered how many other patients had done the same thing and received the same benefit. I began thinking more and more about others who had been through similar surgery and what their experiences had been. I decided to look for written personal accounts. Maryann joined me in searching through libraries and bookstores. We were surprised and disappointed to find no such writings anywhere.

Something else did come from out of the blue, however. Barbara Perler entered the picture.

Advance Therapy

The Perlers lived in Pennsylvania. Barbara's husband Dennis had been a business friend of Richard's for some time. We had been with them on a number of occasions, but not in the past two or three years. Richard somehow learned that Barbara had undergone a brain-tumor operation some months back. When he told me this, I couldn't wait to call her.

Barbara was happy to hear from me, sorry as she was about the coincidence of both of us having developed brain tumors. We began regular telephone conversations that were invaluable to me because of the encouragement I received from them. In no way detracting from the seriousness of brain surgery, she told me things that had a light side to them, things we could laugh about. And laugh we did.

Our talks began with her telling me not to be shocked to see a mummy the first time I looked into a mirror after the operation.

"If you're like I was, you won't be able to see one bit of your head because of the bandages. But it's just as well. This makes it easier to take seeing your bald head when the bandages do come off."

"Bald? You mean your head's shaved?"

"Oh yes, part of it anyway. But that's nothing to worry about. It means you can start being innovative in what you do to hide your head. You'd be surprised at the ideas you can come up with using scarves, and of course, there are wigs."

"What about wigs?"

"You can do a lot with them too. And they become your security. Going out without one can be like going out naked. You can even change your look. One day a blonde, another a brunette, or whatever. Wigs are affordable and easy to care for. Not like the ones available to our mothers. They are lightweight with lots of ventilation and a boost to your morale."

This kind of talk was great for my spirits. There was not the slightest note of concern or fear in anything she said. She had taken some of the mystery out of what I was facing and made it less ominous. What could be more helpful than that? I was glad I had called her. She encouraged me to call her anytime and I took her at her word. Talking to her gave me a wonderful lift.

Avoiding Words

What I learned from the medical encyclopedia helped me to feel well prepared mentally for the operation, and I remained positive about the outcome. But something did get to me more than I should have let it.

By now, virtually everyone with whom we were acquainted had heard about my tumor. This was no surprise. Ours is not a large community and word of this kind gets around in a hurry. What made me conscious of it was the way some people reacted when they saw me.

Normally there would have been some casual conversation, but not now. It was embarrassingly obvious that they wanted to avoid having to talk with me. In the stores they would smile, say a quick hello, then turn away to leave or to occupy themselves with something else. On the street it was much the same – "hello" – and then a hurried exit.

This began disturbing me. I couldn't understand why there should be any change in their feelings toward me. I was the same person as before. I looked the same; there certainly was no exterior sign of the tumor. I had no infectious disease that could be transmitted to anyone else. What was it about my having a brain tumor that would cause some to feel they needed to shun me? It just didn't make sense.

It didn't occur to me that I could be overly sensitive, imagining more than actually was the reality. When I told Richard, he took a much-needed rational view of the whole thing.

"It's just that they don't know what to say, Toni. They probably feel worse about avoiding you than you do about being avoided. They're taking the easy way out. Don't let it bother you. Just think about all the support you have from your close friends. That's more important."

So it was. As I think back now, I knew I was too fearful of being regarded as something other than a normal human being who happened to have a brain tumor that had to be removed. But that stemmed from the negative vision those two frightening words – brain tumor – always seemed to conjure up.

Telling the Truth

By this time, we had told Richard II I was to have an operation on my neck but hadn't made it a serious matter. The main thing we wanted him to know was that I could be in the hospital for a few days. He took it well. He said he was sorry and would miss me, but not to worry about him. Elena would take good care of him.

He was right. Elena had spent a great deal of time with him ever since he was a baby. They were extremely devoted to each other, and we knew he would have the best possible care while I was gone.

It did occur to us, however, that the principal of his school, Dr. Maria Braccia, also should know what the situation was, and I made an appointment with her. She appreciated my concern, and I didn't hold back in telling her about the tumor and the serious nature of the operation.

Dr. Braccia wanted to know just what we had told Richard II about the tumor. From the expression on her face, I could tell she wasn't satisfied with the explanation we had given him.

"You should go much farther than you did and actually use the word tumor," she said. "And you should explain to him just what a tumor is."

"But he's so young," I protested. "We haven't wanted to frighten him."

"It's better that he hear it from you than from other children in the school. And that's bound to happen. Your friends know. Children overhear things at home. Your operation and the reason for it won't be a secret here. Don't expose him to being bewildered and upset by having others tell him what you should tell him yourself."

Of course she was right. Children of our friends and acquaintances were bound to hear about my tumor and the operation I was to have, and naturally there would be talk at school. Richard could hear all sorts of things and be bewildered and hurt that other children knew more about his mother's condition than he himself had been told.

After the talk with Dr. Braccia, we did speak with Richard II again to correct the mistake we had made in not telling him the real story. We told him there was more about my condition that we wanted him to know and our new explanation to him was the same as we had given Susan and Michael. He took it surprisingly well, and we were so relieved to feel we now had done the right thing.

Next, it was Mom's turn to know. She arrived from Florida three days before the operation was to take place. Her friend Chris came with her to our house. Maryann and Dan had arranged for her to stay with them and they would be coming by a little later to get her.

My own positive attitude about the operation was of great help in breaking the news to her. Richard was there, and we told her calmly about the series of events leading up to our meeting with Dr. Fraser and setting the date for the surgery. We assured her we were fully confident of the outcome and didn't want her to worry about it.

Despite our assurances, we knew Mom was shaken by the news. It was inevitable she would be. Knowing her, we could tell that the relative composure she displayed was the opposite of how she felt inside. She sat silent for a few minutes, then asked questions as we talked about the tumor and emphasized how confident we felt that we were in the right hands for the operation. We were glad she showed no resentment that we had waited so long to tell her. She knew, as we did, that she had been spared a lengthy period of worry.

Now that she knew, I had a warm feeling of added security in facing the days ahead. Mom always had been there for Maryann and me to help us through the difficult things. It was comforting to know she was there for me now just as she always had been.

Preparations

There was no shortage of items on my "To Do" lists as the late days of August approached. I was glad to be fully occupied thinking about so many things other than the tumor.

A major assignment, which always called for much discussion, shopping, and compromise, was getting Susan, Michael, and Richard II ready for the reopening of school. It was actually an exciting time, with much going on to get all the bases covered.

As all this was happening, Elena kept assuring me everything concerning the children would go smoothly while I was away. She would see that they were up early, ate breakfast, and got out of the house in time for their school buses. Richard would be with me at the hospital as much as he possibly could be, so it was important for both of us to know everything would be all right at home.

Added assurance came from Maryann and Dan. They would keep in close touch with Elena and the children, check on and help with homework, and make certain there was plenty of weekend activity.

With Elena unable to drive a car, there was a question of who would make the usual frequent trips to the supermarket and other shops for the daily essentials of a family of our size. Jeanie had anticipated I would be worried about this and told me she had arranged things so she could drive Elena wherever she needed to go. Thank goodness for Jeanie. She always was so loyal and helpful.

As for driving the children, Fran, mother of Susan's good friend Devon, would take care of getting Susan wherever she needed to be. And Geri, mother of Michael's friend Dennis, would give Michael and Richard II rides to their various activities. Mom assured me she would be there too. Any "situations" that came up would be handled with loving care by Grandma.

These demonstrations of support and help were so genuine and meaningful that I was touched by them. Yet, they were only among the first of many examples that have helped me through a long period of continuing medical experiences. Never could I emphasize strongly enough the strength that comes from even the smallest of things family and friends do to show how much they truly care.

It was during this period of preparation that I received a telephone call from a woman at the company carrying our health insurance. In accordance with one of their stipulations, it was necessary to notify them in advance of any surgery and hospital stay. This we had done, stating specifically that I would be having brain-tumor surgery and where and when it would be done by Dr. Fraser. So I was dumbfounded at the question she asked me:

"Mrs. Ferrucci, are you sure you have a brain tumor?"

This surprised and annoyed me so much that I gave her a flippant answer.

"Oh, no, we were only kidding when we notified you." There was a brief pause. "If you think I'm lying, recommend a doctor who will tell me I don't have one. I'd be delighted to get the news."

She said it wasn't her job to recommend doctors. Obviously I didn't strike any sense of humor she may possibly have had. And I was sorry to have been that way with her. She was only doing her job, senseless as it seemed to be under the circumstances.

Late August also brought the day Lee had to be in Boulder for his college enrollment. I had been looking forward to going with him and I was excited when the date arrived.

Spring Revisited

Richard found he could get away so both of us could go with Lee to Boulder to help get him set up for his freshman year at the University of Colorado. The trip was to be our luxury for the year, and we looked forward to seeing where Lee would be going to college.

It would be hard to believe any Easterner could visit Colorado without being invigorated by the magnificent mountain scenery and air. We loved what we saw and how we felt from the moment we arrived. We were happy Lee had made this choice of schools.

A friend of Lee's in Garden City, Bryce Carroll, had made the same choice. Bryce's parents, Dan and Ingrid, who were friends of ours, had come to Boulder with him, and we found things we could do together in helping the boys get settled.

The moms tried to help coordinate the room with things the boys had to live with while the dads were put to work figuring out how to make the best use of the smallest space. This was a happy time for me. I was really able to focus on the excitement of this new chapter in Lee's life and put my own problems, at least temporarily, on hold.

From the fun we had helping him, I'm sure we were as excited as Lee about his getting settled in new surroundings.

That evening the Carrolls joined us for dinner at the Flagstaff Restaurant overlooking the city. The view was magnificent. We enjoyed having a dinner in a setting that couldn't have been more lovely.

From our motel, Richard and I had an opportunity to witness a fascinating scene familiar to those who live in an area such as Boulder. Out in the surrounding fields prairie dogs put on their daily show. The little squirrel-like rodents came out of their holes and sat up as if they were in a classroom. We learned that it is a ritual they go through before they begin foraging for food. Seeing this cute exercise was among the many things that made our visit to Colorado a pleasant and memorable one.

Our stay was all too short. When the time approached to leave, Ingrid bet me I would cry when we said goodbye to Lee. I took the bet, sure I could remain composed because he was so happy to be there. She won. When Lee hugged me, told me how much he loved me and said he would pray for me every night, the tears came. Ingrid confessed afterward that she had taken advantage of me. When their oldest son had gone to college, she had cried too.

Another Lesson

The structure of the brain wasn't the only thing I learned about during the days leading to the operation. Though not by choice, I also discovered what double agents steroids can be.

As with most other patients with whom I have shared experiences, the little knowledge I had about steroids was associated with athletes who used them to build strength for competitions. So it was a surprise to have them prescribed to keep my brain from swelling during surgery. This wasn't the end of surprises from these mysterious medications. Soon it was clear that they can extract a heavy price for the benefit they deliver.

Two weeks before the operation date, I began to take the ones that had been prescribed for me. They were tiny, white six-sided pills called Decadron. Knowing how important they must be to the surgery, I made sure to follow carefully the directions for taking them. But I had absolutely no warning of the effects they immediately started to have on me.

All of a sudden I found my joints aching from one end of my body to the other. The persistent discomfort was made worse by inability to sleep at night. No matter how exhausted my body would feel from a busy day, my brain would be wide awake. The only relief: late-night television.

Since I had no idea such side effects would occur, I wondered whether everyone had the same reaction to these particular pills. Surely our pharmacist, Peter, would know and I called him. All he could tell me was that insomnia was a common reaction, but he hadn't been aware of patients suffering from joint aches.

What I wished I had done was find out ahead of time what the side effects might be and whether I could take something else to prevent the brain from swelling but not cause me such difficulties. However, I was to learn later, that there is no effective substitute for the steroids. As many patients can testify, they indeed are a double-edged sword. It is up to the physician to prescribe a dose that hopefully will minimize the side effects while accomplishing the benefit, but total freedom from such problems appears to be rare.

Reflections

Share with Loved Ones

Not long ago, I ran across an anonymous quote in one of my drawers. I've had it for some time, but I don't remember where I got it. How appropriate the words are:

"Trouble is a part of life. And if you don't share it, you don't give the person who loves you enough chance to love you enough."

Richard and I made a mistake in not sharing the truth from the beginning with our three younger children. By thinking we had to protect them, we locked them out from what should have been a family affair all along. A lesson we learned is that it's best to be honest and open with them. Children today are bright at any age. (In fact they probably were in the "old days" too!) They should not be excluded from the facts and left to their own imaginations. Fortunately, we corrected our error, and that brought us closer together. From our children, from other family members, and from close friends, I learned how valuable support and help that come from sharing can be.

Based on my own experience, my strong advice to others in similar situations is to be completely frank from the first diagnosis all the way through to recovery.

A Note to Family and Friends

It is as important for those close to the patient to convey confidence about the operation as it is for the patient to have a positive attitude toward it. Also, if one has business, household, or other responsibilities, there is a need for knowing these will be taken care of during the hospital stay and recovery period. I can testify how much it meant not to have to worry about the children and other things at home.

Reading Material

From what I have been told, Maryann and I did the right thing in going to the library when we wanted to read about brain tumors. The illustrations and explanations in the medical encyclopedia were clear and understandable to lay readers.

Apparently there is a tendency on the part of many patients who want to read about their particular situations to go to medical libraries. This can be a mistake because the material in medical journals can be over the head of many lay persons and can be easily misinterpreted because of that.

Try your public library for one of their standard medical encyclopedias, or ask your doctor or local hospital where you can find one.

Know Your Medications

It is important to know about your medications prescribed at any time. This applies especially to steroids if they are taken in advance of the operation. They can do strange things to the mind and body; it's better to know this before taking them than to have your reactions come as a surprise. It pays to get the answer to four questions:

1. Why am I taking them?
2. For how long?
3. What are the side effects likely to be?
4. How do I deal with those side effects ?

When it was too late, how I wished I had known the answers to those questions ahead of time. Coping with the aftereffects that lingered so long in my body is something I hope never to have to do again. If what I am suggesting here helps to spare others, I'll be happy.

4

Turns in the Road

The Unexpected

For the operation on Thursday, September 12th, I was to enter New York Hospital Tuesday afternoon. It would be a relief to have the waiting end. Painful side effects were constant from almost two weeks of taking the steroids. The aches in my joints never subsided. I tried to get used to them, but didn't fully succeed. Inability to sleep had made watching late-night television a nightly routine. As for the operation itself, I just wanted to get it behind me and be free of that growth pressing on my brain.

Richard stayed home that Tuesday morning and we planned to drive into New York after an early lunch. Everything was ready for my being away. I had managed to keep emotions under control when I said goodbye to Susan, Michael, and Richard II before they left for school. Elena and I had gone over all the things we needed to talk about as far as the household was concerned. I was ready.

Regardless of how well set they may be, how abruptly plans can change. The telephone rang. I answered, thinking it might be Richard's office. Instead, it was Dr. Fraser's secretary. A sudden emergency had arisen with one of his patients. He would not be able to do my operation on Thursday. It would have to be postponed for a week. They were sorry, but the emergency must have priority.

When I hung up the phone and started to think about what this meant, I realized I had mixed emotions. I was disappointed at having to wait but also grateful for the extra time to spend home. The more I thought about it, the more I knew it was only right for the doctor to put an emergency ahead of something less urgent. He had delayed my operation until September at my own request. Another week surely wasn't going to change the outcome. But any delay for the emergency patient probably would be critical. Dr. Fraser deserved to be admired for his decision, and we respected him for doing what he did.

Aside from having to adjust some plans and schedules, the one-week postponement didn't cause any significant upsets for us. I wasn't looking forward to another week of joint aches and insomnia from the steroids I had to keep taking – but I resigned myself to living with them for a few more days. And I easily went back into my normal pattern of driving, shopping, supervising, seeing friends, and all the rest.

When the weekend came, however, I noticed a strange change taking place in my appearance. My face was becoming puffy and round-looking, so much so that I was startled every time I looked at myself in the mirror. As I soon learned, I was developing "moon-face," a common occurrence when certain toxins, in my case the steroids, build up in the system. The condition, aptly called "moon syndrome," can cause the entire body to expand, as it did with me after the operation. I wasn't too happy about having people see me with my face looking that way, but nonetheless, I kept doing things that were normal for me.

It was a great plus to have Mom nearby at Maryann and Dan's. We hadn't seen her since the past Thanksgiving and there was much to talk about. She had kept her youthful outlook on life and lived a busy one in Florida. We talked "a blue streak" when she and Maryann would come over to visit or Mom would come alone but the tumor seldom was mentioned. She told me she was maintaining the same positive attitude I was displaying, and that seemed to suffice for the subject.

Also, there were some visits by friends, and despite my moonface, even an evening out for dinner and to see a movie. The days of the added week slid by and Tuesday came again.

Long Oblivion

This time there was no last-minute change of plans. Richard and I drove into New York early that Tuesday afternoon. Anne Keating had arranged for Richard to spend the night and the next three days in her apartment only blocks from the hospital. It was a great comfort to me to know he would be close throughout the entire operation and would be there beside me when I would waken from it.

After going through the admission procedure at New York Hospital, I was taken to the neurological floor. There I was met by an anesthesiologist. He asked me about any allergies I might have; I wasn't aware of any. He explained how he would administer anesthesia to me for the surgery and said he would be with me all through the operation. I would be asleep and feel nothing at all during the entire time.

The next step was to start on a liquid administered intravenously. This, I was told, would keep me from becoming dehydrated during the several hours of surgery the tumor would require. I remember wanting a bath the morning of the operation. Getting into the tub with this apparatus attached to my arm turned out to be quite a feat, but I was determined because I didn't know when I would be afforded this luxury again!

Immediately after the bath I was wheeled on a stretcher to the operating area. They gave me an extra blanket to keep me warm; operating rooms are always so stark and frigid. Dr. Fraser, wearing a green surgical uniform and cap, greeted me warmly and we had a pleasant brief conversation. He was calm and reassuring, I was confident and ready. Several nurses busied themselves arranging instruments and overhead lights.

Soon I was transferred to the operating table and the anesthesiologist who had talked with me before sat down beside me. It couldn't have been more than a few seconds after I received the anesthetic that I slipped into a deep sleep uninterrupted during the nine straight hours of surgery that followed. The only thing I was vaguely aware of seemed to be a series of unusually bright strobe-like flashes that appeared at some point. They flashed all around me. An explanation for them remains a mystery to this day; apparently no particular significance or meaning could be attached to them. I've asked other brain-surgery patients whether anything similar had happened to them under the anesthesia, but have found no one who had experienced it.

Now Past Tense

I awakened in a recovery room and realized the whole thing was over. What a happy feeling of relief that was. There were bandages wrapped around my head, but I felt no pain. It was hard to believe I had been out for so long. I thought about the bright light flashes, the only things remembered from all those hours. How strange they had been! But the main thing was knowing that the operation was over. I was alive! My brain was working. I had come through intact.

How many of the several hours in the recovery room were spent doing more sleeping, I don't know. I felt drowsy and dosed off frequently. This, I was told, was only normal after the brain's and body's trauma of long, difficult surgery.

When I finally was being wheeled back to my room, I was surprised to see Anne and Len Bullock in the corridor with Richard. They told me later that I greeted them with a big smile and an enthusiastic thumbs-up sign. I can't remember a bit of it but I'm sure that was true. The joy in knowing the operation was over, combined with seeing them there, did give me precisely that kind of feeling.

The Bullocks, close friends for years, had flown up that morning from their home in Charlotte, North Carolina, to be with Richard throughout the day and with me, when I came out of recovery. Anne had been through serious surgery the year before and felt she could be of help to me in the early stages of my recuperation. I was delighted to have her there, as well as Len, and Richard surely was appreciative of their being with him.

The next day I discovered that an aftermath of the operation was causing great concern. Different doctors began coming in and going out of my room. They were worried about my right eye. It had vision, but decreased mobility. Apparently a nerve had been unavoidably damaged in making a pathway to the tumor. Although I could see, the eye couldn't move from left to right. The conclusion was that nothing could be done about it, but since nerves can repair themselves, there was hope the nerve eventually would come back to life. Naturally I was distressed, but tried to think of the situation in a positive way. If the nerve *could* come back, it *would* come back.

The hospital stay was one week. Richard came for long visits every day and his being there was wonderful therapy for me. Anne Keating came, frequently with her sister Dodie who also lived in New York. They were great company and it always gave me a lift when they walked through the doorway, alone or together.

Some friends came in from Garden City but their visits were shorter than I would have liked because I would get so tired. Richard and I talked about his bringing the children in, but since I would be home in a few days, we decided to have my reunion with them there.

The bandages remained on my head for a time. None of us could guess how I would look when they were removed. We were in for both shock and surprise. One thing I did know for sure, there was another problem with my right eye. I had double vision. I began learning how to compensate for it by keeping the eye closed when I wanted to see things clearly. By no means, though, was I accepting the condition as permanent; I kept telling myself nerves can repair themselves. I was thankful there had been no perceptible loss of hearing, but I was conscious of definite numbness in the right side of my face. This too was nerve damage and could repair itself.

Back Home

My release from the hospital on Thursday, September 26th, was in mid-afternoon and we drove home in the usual heavy Long Island traffic. By then, the bandages had been removed, but I hadn't seen myself in a mirror. One of the nurses had wrapped a scarf around my head and I wouldn't know what was under it until later.

It was late in the afternoon by the time we arrived at our house – and what a thrill it was to be back! Susan, Michael, and Richard II were there. They had made welcome home signs and placed them at locations I would have to pass wherever I went. In addition they had helped Elena decorate the dinner table festively for my homecoming. It was all so touching that I cried as I hugged each one of them and felt the warmth being expressed to me.

At the same time I was aware of surprised stares, first my own, after I stepped into the downstairs powder room and removed the scarf. What I immediately noticed in the mirror was the peculiar position of my right eye, as if it somehow had turned on its side. Then the head. What a shock! The right side was shaved, but a funny little flap had been left on top. There in the middle of the baldness was a large scar in the shape of a question mark. I never thought I could look so awful. I was embarrassed about having the children see me.

It was amusing, however, to hear Michael's reaction. He said I could dye the hair on the left side blue and be in real fashion as a "punk rocker." When I tried putting the scarf on again to hide the big scar, Richard II wanted to know what I was doing. When I told him I thought I looked funny and was trying to do something about it, he said I never could look funny to him. I could have given him the world for saying something that made me feel so good. As for Susan, she seemed to be having a hard time adjusting to my appearance; it obviously was beyond what she had expected.

This was the first sign of growing awareness by the children that the full story about the operation had been kept from them. For along with the affected eye, the big scar, and rigidness in the right side of my face, there was continuing "moon syndrome" with the puffed face and expanded body. Logically, all these changes wouldn't have resulted from a simple operation on the neck to remove a tumor that had grown at the base of the brain, as the operation had been pictured to them.

Strange Happenings

The immediately visible effects the children became aware of were joined by other aftermaths I certainly hadn't anticipated. As explained to me, three influences had converged to set them in motion: (1) disturbances to the brain by the operation, (2) adverse reactions as a result of taking steroids for three weeks, and (3) metabolic (chemical) reaction to medications administered at the hospital. This combination was in the process of bringing me the weirdest "spaced-out" sensations. In addition to these were an occasional feeling of being scared and not knowing why, a diminished attention span, and frustrating memory lapses. All this plus an insatiable craving for sweets which had started in the hospital.

Conscious as I was of these disturbing developments, I was so busy those first few days that I managed to keep them from interfering with what I was doing.

Mom had been able to stay long enough for me to be back home and I was particularly happy about this.

We spent some wonderful time together before she had to return to Florida. It meant so much to me to know she was there during the whole period of the operation. It had to be an anxious, worrisome time for her and I was thankful she had been so strong and seemingly calm in going through it.

Richard's mother Jo came down from Connecticut and stayed overnight the following Sunday. It was the first time we had seen her since considerably before the operation. As mentioned earlier, we purposely had kept it from her. She was terribly angry and upset about our having been so unfair to her. We were just as sorry she was upset, but felt the best course was the one we had followed.

With visits from my good friends, there was constant activity in the house those first few days. There were so many cards to acknowledge; these cards had loving messages that made me more and more conscious of how much warm, caring friendships can mean and how fortunate I was to have them.

Even though I was busy, I couldn't escape my concern about the aftereffects of the surgery. I kept wondering how long I would have to cope with them. In no way, however, was I expecting the new episodes that began occurring out of the blue and soon had me back in New York Hospital.

Jeanie and I had gone shopping in Cedarhurst, not far from Garden City. We had stopped to look at clothes in the window of one of the stores along the main business street. Without warning, the entire left side of my body seemed to collapse and I began falling toward the glass. Jeanie's instantaneous reaction, perfected by experiences in holding out an arm to secure a child in the days before car seat belts, was to reach out and grab me before I fell into that window.

It was so quick and such a close call that I was totally unnerved for the moment. Jeanie held me tightly as we walked into the store and found a chair. The expressions on the faces of the salespeople changed quickly when Jeanie explained that I recently had a brain operation. I was glad they got the truth. Until then, they probably thought I had one too many drinks at lunch.

That ended our shopping tour for the day. We didn't want a repetition of the episode, so headed home. It was good we did. The same thing struck me again the next morning at home, as well as later that afternoon. It was a sensation of sudden numbness moving completely through my leg, causing it to collapse under me. With no control and a feeling of utter helplessness, down I would go in an embarrassing heap. Luckily, I wasn't hurt, but this was something scary that couldn't go on. We had no idea of what possibly could be wrong; whatever it was, we knew we had better find out in a hurry.

An Addition

An anxious call to Dr. Fraser produced an answer. Fluid had built up in my brain. The extra fluid, accumulating at and around the surgical area, naturally would have an effect if it began pressuring vital adjacent areas. In my case, this had happened.

Because of the urgency of draining the fluid, Dr. Fraser set the morning of October 4th as the date for another operation. The purpose this time was to insert a shunt, a procedure I understood to be normal under such circumstances. The thought of having a foreign object in my brain didn't disturb me if it would get rid of those sudden collapses. It would be a simple operation compared with the first.

My stay at New York Hospital this time was four days. The shunt was explained to me as consisting of two flexible tubes (catheters) and a valve. One of the tubes is inserted at the best location inside the brain to capture and drain the excess fluid that builds up. A valve is attached to this to prevent backflow. The second tube, attached to and leading from the valve, is inserted down through the chest and into the abdomen for the fluid to be absorbed by normal body action.

This operation posed no difficulties for me. Dr. Fraser commented that I had tolerated the procedure well and showed no signs of complications. So on I went to a recovery room with a tremendous feeling of relief. I could now get on with dealing with the other lingering effects.

The shunt was something I had to get used to. There was no way to avoid being conscious of its presence. After all, it was an addition, not only to my brain, but to the upper part of my body. And I would have it all my life. This would be no ordeal though. The purpose it was serving was so essential that I must, and would, accept the ingenious object as a fact of life.

When I arrived home from the hospital this time, I was pleased with how good I actually felt. The other aftereffects still had to be dealt with, of course. And the only way to do that, I knew, was to be determined to get them behind me as soon as possible.

On with Life

It was inevitable that the obviousness of continuing effects from the tumor surgery, awareness of my collapses, and my having to go back to the hospital for the shunt would surprise and also alarm Susan and Michael. We had wanted to spare them concern and worry about my tumor, but apparently we had gone too far. I remember so vividly what Susan said shortly after I came back from the second New York Hospital stay:

"We thought it was a tumor in the neck that happened to be at the brainstem. We didn't know it really was a tumor on the brain. Naturally we would think it was something that would be easy to remove – no big operation. Now we know it was just the opposite. Why didn't you tell us? We're part of the family. We love you. We want to know when something is wrong. We want to help."

Michael fully agreed with her. He said there were so many things he would have wanted to do for me if he had known the full truth about my tumor and how serious it was. He felt even Richard II probably had known more than he and Susan had.

It was hard to defend having told them only part of the story. Our intentions surely had been good. But we had followed the wrong route in not going the full distance with them. What it all came down to was that we had underestimated the ability of our own children, young as they were, to be able to hear the truth, understand the truth, and deal with it intelligently. We promised that from then on, they would know everything we knew about my situation. And I think we've lived up to that promise.

Meanwhile, I was hoping to get back to as normal a pattern of living as possible while coping with the changes in my life. And over the next few weeks I made some progress in doing so.

Driving, for example. I found I could do it safely despite my affected right eye. My peripheral vision was not good and I learned to compensate by making maximum use of the side view mirrors. I didn't attempt to drive at night, however, because in the dark it was a different story. But the fact I could get around during the day meant I could go shopping, and do other errands.

One thing I must admit is that I did find an excuse for not doing much cooking, leaving that chore mainly to Elena. After one of my ongoing telephone conversations with Barbara Perler, I just had to have a new wig for trying some things she suggested. Jeanie went with me to look for it and we had fun shopping for the right one. When we found it and the salesman was writing up the transaction, he warned me about something:

"Keep in mind that these wigs are flammable. Don't get too close to flames or hot electric burners."

In assuring him I would be careful, I found a great excuse for staying away from the kitchen stove. (This didn't bother me at all! I had never had a flair for cooking the way Maryann and Jeanie did.)

That wig really did things for me. Richard II was playing in a soccer game the Saturday after I bought it. His father, knowing how much it would mean if he were to go to see the game, was surprised when I said I would join him. I *did* and even stayed the whole game. The wig looked very much like my own hair; wearing it, I felt I could face the world. So I truly enjoyed the game, and it was a great boost for my morale.

As for the continuing aftereffects, it was apparent they were going to remain for a long while. Dr. Fraser had suggested that I enroll in a therapy program with exercises to strengthen my weak left side. For a short time, I even went with Nora Forelli to the therapist to whom she was going for a problem with her shoulder. This made me aware of the importance of exercises to help heal my body, but I decided to do them at home.

Another Operation?

Although Richard had told me at the hospital after the September 19th surgery that another operation might be necessary, I somehow must have blocked it from my memory. Or maybe I used selective memory and only recorded things I wanted to hear. For I had then and still have absolutely no recollection of it. Yet, I know Richard's memory, and when he said he had told me, I knew it must have been true.

The tumor was so hard and resistant and in such a vulnerable location that despite nine hours of intensive surgery, Dr. Fraser had been able to remove only a part of it. In discussing this with Richard, he had suggested waiting for a follow-up MRI after mid-October to consider what the next step might be.

It was now time for that follow-up MRI, and we scheduled it at a local radiological office. The results would be dispatched to Dr. Fraser who then would be in touch with us.

So, when I went for the imaging that October day, I had no idea of what the actual situation was. In no way was I prepared for news that came in a conversation Richard had with Dr. Fraser a few days later. He told Richard that because so much of the tumor remained, another operation should be scheduled, but he felt it best to wait until spring. This would provide time for me to recover from what I already had been through. Since the tumor was not now exerting pressure on the brain, there was no reason for doing it sooner.

The totally unexpected prospect of another operation came as a real blow to me. Going through all of it again was the last thing I wanted to do. I did not feel sure I would be up to doing it. My immediate reaction was to think back about what I had read in the library medical encyclopedia on my type of tumor. It was slow growing because it was not the aggressive kind. Wasn't there a possibility it had been reduced in size at least enough to eliminate danger? Wasn't it even possible the surgery could have stopped its growth?

Wishes. Hopes. Dreams. But worth clinging to. It was October. Spring was months away. Anything was possible. I had to get on with my life now. Another operation might be inevitable but brooding about it would accomplish nothing. There were too many positive things to think about with the holiday season ahead. Better to concentrate on them.

Reflections

Stay Busy

A necessity while waiting for the operation, once it is scheduled, is to keep your mind as fully occupied as possible. Patients with whom I have talked agree it is wise to find other things to think about. If there are too many idle hours, they can turn into worry sessions. Even after I began having effects from the steroids before my first operation, I tried to stay with my usual busy schedule.

The same is true when there are many aftereffects, as in my case, and a long period of time is needed to deal with them. There were many times during the night when it was extremely hard to suppress concern about ever really being normal again. For such times, I had an antidote, late night television. During the day I did all I could to keep myself occupied with a full schedule of normal activity. Regardless of what they may be, having things to keep the mind busy is tremendously important.

A Plea

There is a tendency to look upon a brain-tumor patient as somehow different after the operation. I know this from little things I observed and heard over the weeks following my return home. Other patients have told me they've had the same experience.

Except for having had the surgery and perhaps requiring follow-up therapy, the person taken into the operating room has not been transformed into some other form of human being before being brought back out. It is essential to the patient's morale to be regarded as the same person he/she always has been.

5

Making Adjustments

Needing Help

Getting over the continuing problems I was having with effects from the tumor surgery was my main concern as I thought about the approaching holiday season. There seemed to be little progress, and I was anxious to find ways of getting rid of them faster than just letting nature take its course.

The episodes of feeling "spaced out" were especially disturbing. Not only would I have the sensation that my mind was off somewhere away from my body, but I was told my voice sounded as if I had inhaled laughing gas. And although I felt my mind was somewhere in space, I was fully conscious of things going on around me. I really didn't care what was happening, though; it was as if I somehow were detached from reality.

When my mind would come back to me and things seemed normal again, I would think, even hope, I had been through a dream, nothing more. From others who had been with me, however, I found out what actually had happened, how truly spaced out I had been. And I was sure these episodes had something to do with a strange fear that sometimes would grip me – the feeling of being afraid and not knowing why.

My diminished attention span and the related difficulties I had remembering things added to my worry. I knew my memory was affected, but didn't realize until sometime later how really bad it had become. I couldn't remember where I had put things, where my things were kept, what clothes I had worn the day before, even what I might have said or done an hour before. The children were most disturbed about these lapses. They would tell me things and I would have absolutely no recollection of them. I guess sometimes I would get so completely frustrated when my mind went blank that I would sit in silence and just stare with an angry look on my face at the floor or the wall or whoever might be nearby. Poor Elena! This happened several times when the two of us were in the same room doing something. She thought I was angry with her and couldn't understand why. She was so hurt that she finally asked me what she had done to make me so unhappy with her. I was totally surprised.

"Elena, I'm not angry with you. You've done absolutely nothing to make me unhappy." I reached out my arms to her. "I love you, Elena. We all love you."

Her tears as we hugged each other were from the relief and comfort of knowing my angry stares weren't directed at her. She now understood they were part of the condition I was undergoing and hopefully would soon overcome.

Another aspect of it certainly out of character for me was a pronounced loss of confidence in my ability to do things that normally had been routine. This extended to such simple matters as deciding what we should have for dinner. And it made me reluctant to leave the security of the house. I was afraid to accept certain invitations because I wasn't sure I could find my way, especially to places unfamiliar to me. In order to go, I had to have exact directions, block by block, turn by turn.

This loss of confidence led me to begin leaning heavily on Maryann to help with decisions about the children, their activities, and their constant requests to do things and go places. And when Mom arrived from Florida to be with us through Thanksgiving, I began relying on her to do things I normally would have done.

The fact my memory had been affected caused simple decisions to become magnified into overwhelming situations I had trouble dealing with. This couldn't go on. From what I had been told, time would be the healer, and these disturbing, disruptive things eventually would be behind me. But I decided it was up to me to take hold of myself and help time do the healing.

Plain, simple logic pointed to two keys and I had to use both of them. One, I must really work at getting back my mind's stability and my memory's sharpness by trying harder and harder to think about and concentrate on everything I did. Two, it was essential for me to get into some kind of routine that would be effective in helping my brain and my body to overcome the continuing effects and get back to normal.

Advice and Action

A close family friend, Gary Giulietti, had made quite a study of ways to keep the body in top shape. He put into practice things he learned and figured out for himself. His energy, enthusiasm, and splendid physical condition were convincing evidence that his theories and ideas worked. And he seemed pleased when I asked his advice on what I should do.

From then on he was my "coach." He set out a plan for me, a simple routine. I was to drink a great deal of water, as much as I thought I could tolerate and then more. The idea was to increase the rate at which the disturbing substances remaining in my blood and tissues would be eliminated from my brain and body. Also I was to begin a program of more serious exercise than what I had been doing. This would involve daily walking. In addition, I was to take three kinds of vitamins – A, C and E – as well as the trace element (mineral) selenium.

Gary reasoned that these combined steps not only would help me with the other problems, but also help me to get back to normal body size. The moon syndrome that had expanded my face and entire body was a great embarrassment to me; how happy I would be when I no longer felt and looked like a blimp! I realized, though, that I had to do more to help and that meant curbing my appetite for sweets. The actual cravings had diminished as I discontinued steroids, but I had developed a "habit" of grabbing whatever was easiest – usually something sweet.

I'm sure my inflated body drew many comments that I never knew about, but there was one in particular that still genuinely amuses me when I think back to that first year. It was shortly before Lee arrived home from college for Thanksgiving. His friend Rich Forelli already was back from school and came over to see me. He and Lee talked after that and Lee asked him how I was. This, we learned later and with much laughing, was his reply:

"She's great, but she looks like the Pillsbury Doughboy."

Rich's description, appropriate as it was, became quite a joke with us. And, believe me, it's good to have some things you can laugh about when going through a long period of recovery. They help to reduce the tension that easily can build up when gains seem dishearteningly slow. How many times I said to myself, "I'm all right. I can still laugh. And as long as I can do that, I can get where I'm going."

Diversions

Along with laughs, there were many things that helped me keep a positive mental attitude.

For one, Jeanie and I kept affirming how right Barbara Perler had been when she talked about the joys of wigs. We would do the rounds of the wig stores, and we really did have fun. We would try on those named for celebrities – Barbra Streisand, Diana Ross, Cher – and end up trying others we thought fitted our own personalities. Actually, I wanted to look as close as possible to the way I looked before the operation. That wasn't easy with my puffed face; I was expecting a lot from a wig.

Richard was with us on one of our trips to the wig shops, and he really got into the spirit of things. He had me trying all sorts of more daring looks. I think he thought it would be exciting after 21 years of marriage to have a "new" wife. I'm afraid I spoiled his fantasy by wanting to stay the way I was – without the moonface, of course.

Mom and I had some fun times, too. She usually came north to be with us for Thanksgiving, and it was especially wonderful for me to have her that year. As always we had endless things to talk about, and we would find many excuses to get out of the house. One day, I remember, we drove out east beyond Riverhead to a favorite fruit and vegetable stand. We had discovered it years before and tried always to make at least one trip there every fall. We laughed as we drove home with the car packed with goodies. Now we had to make sure we hid them from the kids so that we had at least a few things left by the time Thanksgiving rolled around.

Thanksgiving dinner would be festive as always. Along with Mom being there, Richard's mother Jo and brother Tony would come down from Connecticut. Maryann and Dan would be joining us, with Maryann, a true expert with food, preparing and bringing some of the dishes that would look as delicious as they would taste. And Mom would have an active hand in the preparations also. Every year it was a busy kitchen reminiscent of Thanksgivings of times past.

As for blessings, we always counted them on this day of family gathering and feasting. As I considered them at church that morning, something almost miracle-like happened. I could tell that my mind was totally obliterating any thoughts of negatives. I would spend the day enjoying and being grateful for the blessings of life and of love.

Assessing Progress

With the holiday having come and gone, it was back to reality in facing and trying to deal with the stubborn effects that persisted in afflicting me. Although I had started doing the things Gary had prescribed, I hadn't really followed through over the Thanksgiving holiday. Now I knew I had to get into a daily routine and stay with it.

At some points, I had felt the spaced-out episodes were less intense, but soon realized this must have been more wish than fact; they really hadn't changed. I had gone to work on my memory by trying harder to con-centrate. This would work, I was sure, but I had a long, long way to go. I had kept looking in the mirror and thinking maybe my blimp-like body was showing signs of thinning, but I wasn't sure I could trust my own judgment. Occasional tingling in the right side of my face kept me hoping life was returning.

Something else I had to do was find out what could be done about my right eye that couldn't move.

Dr. Michael Slavin, a neurological ophthalmologist at Long Island Jewish Medical Center was highly recommended to me. I was able to get an appointment with him and was impressed with the way he examined my eye, analyzed its condition, and suggested what could be done about it.

He explained that the nerve which controls eye movement had been damaged in the operation. This had caused restriction in the muscle that performs the movement action in response to the nerve. Fairly recently, medical research has found that botulinum toxin (botox), mainly associated with serious effects from contaminated food, has a positive side to it. Used neurologically in small doses, it can relax and help certain impaired muscles, including those in the eye, to balance movement.

Dr. Slavin went on to point out that long-term correction of the condition would depend on the nerve's repairing itself over a period of time. An injection of botulinum toxin could bring relief for the immediate future, however, and he felt it desirable to take this step. He wanted to have another opinion, though, and sent me to Dr. Steven Rubin, a pediatric ophthalmologist at North Shore University Hospital. This specialist, well experienced in botulinum injections, agreed that this step was appropriate.

Dr. Rubin, under the watchful eye of Dr. Slavin, proceeded a short time later with the injection. It did achieve the purpose of restoring movement in the eye, even though I still had double vision. I was glad I had found these two doctors whom I liked a great deal.

A Different Christmas

Although I was driving and doing other things I had done before, I was by no means close to being "back to normal" in my activities. Due in part to the continuing aftereffects, I frequently was tired, almost worn out, and just didn't have the energy to do everything I felt I should do and really wanted to do.

Having to recognize that fact filled me with anxiety about the approaching Christmas. It was a special time at our house. I always had enjoyed getting ready for it – shopping, decorating, baking, all the other things that made it such a joyous season of the year. Would I be able to do them this time? No – I had to tell myself that I just wasn't up to all of it, no matter how much I might push myself to extend my capabilities.

What happened out of the blue came as such a wonderful solution that I called it then and still think of it as our Christmas miracle of 1991.

Carolyn Casano telephoned one evening and said she and Charlie wanted to come right over to tell us something exciting. She wouldn't give me a clue as to what it was; we would have to wait until they arrived.

Carolyn was right when she had used the word exciting. Some good friends of theirs had a lodge out in Vail, Colorado. They wouldn't be using it until New Year's Day. They had offered it to the Casanos for a skiing vacation over Christmas. And their place was large enough that the Casanos could bring another family if they wished. Charlie, Carolyn and the Casano children, the same ages as ours, wanted us to be the other family. What great friends they always have been!

Christmas away from home. Would it be right for the children? As the four of us talked about it that evening, we decided it actually could be more fun for them than the usual routine of Christmas Day. Moreover, if we made our reservations right away, we could get special reduced airline fares that would make the trip reasonable. So, it could be everyone's Christmas gift.

It would be a very special Christmas. Susan and Richard II were sorry we wouldn't have our annual Christmas tree; other than that, they were happy and excited. Michael, an excellent skier, thought it would be the best way he could spend Christmas. Lee, who would join us from Boulder, was thrilled we were coming to Colorado. As for Richard and me, we both felt it would be a happy time.

It was indeed a very special holiday. Our six days in Vail were delightful for all of us. Although I didn't do any skiing, I was occupied and invigorated just being there in such a beautiful setting. And what fun evenings we had. Watching *Jeopardy* on television had become a ritual with me and I didn't want to give it up just because we weren't home. So all of us took to watching the nightly show. When I had a particularly "knowledgeable" evening, Carolyn said she knew I had something taken out of my brain but how did I get them to insert all these facts?

Our Christmas miracle of 1991 – a miracle made possible by loving friendships.

Thoughts Ahead

The last day of that fateful 1991 is one I remember particularly well because of the confusion of emotions it brought me.

Things went well until mid-afternoon. I had done some shopping in the morning and had driven Susan, Michael, and Richard II to various places. Maryann had come over for lunch and she, Lee and I had a very pleasant talk about his work at college. It was when I went upstairs a little later to have a short rest that one of my spaced-out episodes took over. I had thought these were getting less severe, but this one seemed especially intense.

A question I had tried and pretty much succeeded in keeping submerged forced itself out as I moved my head back and forth trying to shake off the fuzziness:

"Am I ever going to be normal again?"

So many weeks had gone by since the operation. I was following the program Gary had designed for me. In many respects, I was back to normal. Yet, these outer-space sensations still came without warning. My memory was still uncertain all too many times. Double vision still bothered me, though I had learned to compensate for it. And while I had lost a little weight, it was so painfully slow that I had to wonder whether all the excess would ever go away.

Richard and Gary kept reminding me that I had to be patient. They said they could see little improvements that I probably was hardly aware of because I was anxious for big improvements. They undoubtedly were right, but the beginning of a new year with those negative effects was far from a bright one. And that wasn't all.

Much as I had avoided thinking about it, there was the lurking prospect of another operation. Dr. Fraser had said it could wait until spring. Spring would arrive before we knew it. Would I face a repetition of the whole process? The possibility of this would make anyone apprehensive.

So, there was little wonder that my mood was melancholy as I thought about the new year. The fact January 1st also was my birthday didn't help to make matters any brighter. There would be "Happy Birthday" wishes throughout the day. But the recipient wouldn't be very happy.

Richard and I planned a quiet New Year's Eve. Except for Lee, who was going to a party, we would take the children out to dinner. Then we would come home, watch television later, and wait for the annual Times Square ball to drop, ushering in 1992.

At dinner we had so many things to talk about, including our Colorado vacation. Back home, Richard and I busied ourselves with "Happy New Year" telephone calls. It was well after 11:00 o'clock when we sat down to watch television during 1991's final hour.

My mind really wasn't on what was flickering across the screen. It was on the changes in my life the year had brought me, the totally unexpected events set in motion by finding out what caused my recurring neck pain. It was a year I certainly didn't want to repeat. Yet, there was a very real possibility that this was precisely what I would have to do.

Still, wasn't there another consideration? The things I had thought about back in October when I learned about the prospect of a second operation. The possibility that enough of the tumor had been removed to eliminate danger of pressure on vital parts of the brain. The possibility that the surgery had stopped the tumor's growth. With a new year at hand, wasn't it the time to hold hope for good things?

By midnight, my positive attitude had reasserted itself. The year 1992 could be a good one. An end to aftereffects from the operation. No new operation. A year of being back as a normal human being.

Yes, of course. I became more and more optimistic. The thought of a wonderful way to keep myself fully occupied during the early part of the year began forming. There couldn't be another operation in the spring. I would have too much to do. And the disturbing effects would have to end; I wouldn't have time for coping with them.

Midnight. Richard was elated with my exhilaration as we kissed to welcome 1992 – and my birthday.

Reflections

A Desired Virtue

For me, it was difficult not to get discouraged and frustrated in trying to cope with aftereffects of the operation that plagued me for so long. I realized how important it was to have patience, but acquiring and maintaining this desirable virtue wasn't easy.

What helped the most to carry me through was assurance from those whose judgment I respected that eventually I would get over the problems and be my normal self again.

With this assurance, I found I could be more certain in my own mind about achieving my goals. And that certainly strengthened my determination, however long and slow the process might be.

The key, then, is to know not only that recovery from lingering effects *can* occur, but that it *will* occur if you are determined and persistent.

Needed Help

Despite the most extraordinary care taken by the surgeon, it is virtually impossible to penetrate the brain without disturbing vital nerves. Although they will recover from minor injury, this can take time.

Logically, nerves resist added work until they have recovered sufficiently to begin taking it on again.

Resistance to making decisions appears to be high on the list of aftereffects. For me, this extended to losing confidence in my ability to make simple decisions.

In this situation, there is a message for family and friends. Don't push the patient's brain to do this added work until willingness and capability are clearly evident. The brain needs time to get over the trauma it has undergone.

6

A Long Reprieve

A Good Start

Following the October operation I had been advised to see a neurologist on a regular basis to check for any possible symptoms of tumor recurrence. In the spring, then, I was to have another MRI to see what the pictures would show.

In November and December, I had gone to a neurologist in New York. The trip back and forth to the city was one I didn't relish, however, and it became apparent that it would be better for me to have a doctor on Long Island.

My good fortune was to have a friend recommend Dr. Alan Mazurek whose office was in Rockville Centre, just 15 minutes from Garden City. My first appointment with him was on January 2nd of the new year. I immediately liked him and felt relieved that I could see him regularly by going a short distance, or if the need should arise, on short notice.

Dr. Mazurek told me that I should have an MRI in the spring and one every six months after that. I was happy with the clear implication in this that there would be no new operation in the spring, as Dr. Fraser initially had suggested. From what I learned, Dr. Fraser thought he had cut off the blood supply to the tumor when he performed the long, difficult surgery. This could mean there would be no further growth unless in some way the tumor could reattach itself to a source of blood. That would remain to be seen; thus the importance of follow-up MRIs.

Dr. Mazurek was thorough in asking me questions about effects I was still experiencing from the October operation. He was pleased with the condition of my eye and confirmed that nerves can repair themselves, but that it would take time. So there was hope; I had to be patient. As to the spaced-out episodes, my uncertain memory, the scared feeling without knowing why that sometimes came over me, and the moon syndrome, it was still a matter of patience. They gradually would go away. And feeling eventually could return to the numb side of my face.

Encouraged by my discussion with this fine doctor, I told Gary about it. He was pleased I had had such a talk and reemphasized the need for carefully following the program he had given me: drinking lots of water, exercising consistently, and taking the prescribed vitamins. All this was in my power and I was determined to do it.

The following Saturday, January 4th, Jeanie had a surprise birthday luncheon for me. She had invited Maryann and several of my close friends. It was wonderful to be with them to start the new year. I was feeling more and more confident it would be a good one. And I told them about an idea that had begun forming in my mind on New Year's Eve.

In April, Richard would turn 50 and Michael 16. Why not a surprise party for the two of them? Our father, who always had been generous with Maryann and me, had left each of us some money to be used for something special. The combined birthday party could be the kind of special thing he had in mind. And I knew that preparing for it would be good therapy for me. The girls at the luncheon loved the idea and all volunteered to help. It would be fun – a group project. Right then and there we began talking about plans for it.

Steady Progress

Richard kept reminding me about needing patience to deal with continuing effects. I found, however, that patience is not an easy virtue to come by when disturbing aftereffects are so relentless for so long. That's why, I began calling in earnest on another source of help: my faith.

This was not the first time I had done so since learning I had the tumor. From the very outset, I had prayed for positive thinking and the ability to handle whatever might lie ahead. And I remember so well how reciting two rosaries kept me calm through my first

MRI; Susan had bought me wooden beads at St. Patrick's Cathedral on one of her trips to Manhattan. I was able to bring them into the machine since no metal was allowed, and they have been with me for all the MRIs since.

The fact is that throughout my long series of medical experiences I have felt a spiritual presence by my side. For this I have been grateful to ever so many who have prayed for me to come through the operations successfully and to be in good health. These have included not only family and friends, but three priests to whom Richard and I have been devoted for their friendship. Two of them, Charles Swiger and Joseph Murray, are pastors at Long Island churches. Monsignor Swiger's visits and blessings gave me needed strength. And I'll never forget what Father Murray said to me before my second set of operations: "I'm storming Heaven with prayers for you." The third, Vincent Hagen, a parish priest I got to know in Garden City, has since been transferred to Canada and writes frequently. He visits me with words of continued encouragement on any of his trips to our area.

Since it was plain I had to be patient about overcoming the clinging aftereffects, I began praying for the discipline needed to keep from being irritated and frustrated by the painfully slow pace of recovery. Prayers helped me have the confidence that there would be progressive improvement.

Meanwhile, plans were beginning to take shape for the big dual birthday party scheduled for April 11th.

Even as far in advance as January, we were getting excited about it. Arrangements were made to hold it in one of the party rooms at the Garden City Hotel. We were talking about food to discuss with the caterer and about decorations to have in the room. Every day we were adding names to the list of friends to invite. The one thing worrying us was, with all the preparations that would be going on and more and more persons knowing about the party, could we keep it a secret from Richard and Michael.

The birthday celebration wasn't my sole preoccu-pation by any means, but it did prove to be a great morale builder for me. I know that the planning generated along the way, combined with the other positive influences, brought about a noticeable, steady decline in the negatives produced by the toxins that stayed so long in my body.

Miraculously, thanks to all the people we pledged to secrecy, the day of the party arrived without Richard or Michael being aware of what was going to happen that evening. Later I found out Michael thought we were going for a family dinner to celebrate Richard's birthday, and Richard assumed there would probably be two or three other couples to surprise him for his upcoming 50th.

Things had come a long way since January. I hadn't had the MRI yet; Dr. Mazurek had agreed to put it off until after the party. It wasn't that I was afraid of the possibility of bad news; it was just that I didn't want to take the slightest chance of anything marring the birthday celebration.

As for the operation's aftereffects that had been such a problem, I really had worked at overcoming them and there had been much progress. The day of the party I took stock of each of them. I remember the exact list I made in my mind:

- *The episodes of being spaced out.* Mostly gone. Only an occasional one, and this much less severe than they had been before.

- *Memory lapses.* Still a problem, but considerable improvement. Continuing need for patience and concentration to be certain of things.

- *Strange sensations of being afraid and not knowing why.* Still a mystery, but no longer having them.

- *Craving for sweets.* I missed them, but was glad to have lost my insatiable appetite for them.

- *Moon syndrome.* Although I was still a bit on the heavy side, I no longer had that blimp-like appearance.

- *Double vision.* This had stayed with me. I had become well practiced in keeping the right eye closed and making head movements to increase the range of vision in the good left eye. By no means had I given up, however, on thinking and hoping that one day the eye itself would correct the condition.

- *Numbness on the right side of my face.* Still present. Again, though, I had not stopped holding onto the thought and hope that some day the occasional tingling would turn into full sensation.

Everything considered, there had been marked improvements in the early months of 1992. I was pleased, so were Richard, the children, and my friends. I really had come a long way.

Spring Imaging

The birthday party was a wonderful success. Richard and Michael were genuinely surprised and overwhelmed when they entered the room, and saw so many people there – adult friends of Richard's, young friends of Michael's – and heard "Happy Birthday" sung to each of them. Everything turned out just right. It was a never-to-be forgotten evening, and it made me so happy that I couldn't give enough praise to the friends who worked with me to put the affair together. There was no way I could have done it without them. And I couldn't have been more grateful to my father for that special fund he left me to be used for just such a purpose.

With the party over, I now had to get to the reality of scheduling an MRI. Dr. Mazurek suggested an imaging center not far from his office.

From the time of the October operation, I had had no symptoms or signals to indicate that the tumor was active in any degree. The hope was that it had become dormant for lack of blood supply and would remain that way. For apparently enough of it had been removed to keep it from pressing adjacent areas or nerves. So, if there were no further growth, it could be left alone. I would know it was there, but could live with that, if it were dormant.

All this of course was speculation. We wouldn't know how true it might be until the MRI had looked inside to find out. Carrying my wooden rosary beads, I approached the cylinder with inner confidence about what it would reveal.

Dr. Mazurek called the next day to give me the results. He said there appeared to have been no growth in the tumor, at least as nearly as could be determined from looking at the pictures. Though much of it remained intact, it apparently wasn't creating pressure. Since it wasn't causing me problems, there was no urgency about another operation. However, he strongly recommended that I make an appointment to see Dr. Fraser and get his interpretation of the MRI.

We saw Dr. Fraser and he concurred with Dr. Mazurek's reading, but reminded us, "there's no free lunch."

Overall, this was good news for the time being and I was pleased. But it did imply that the possibility of another operation would hang over my head from one MRI to the next, not a happy prospect. Off and on for the rest of the day I thought about this and how to handle it.

Realistically, there was no way I was going to be able to block that prospect totally from my mind for six months at a time. The last thing in the world I wanted to do, though, was brood about it at any point along the way. The only sensible course was to live my life as if nothing were going to happen after any of those MRIs. If by chance something negative should show up at some future time, I would deal with it then; there was nothing to be gained in anticipating what it would mean and what I would do about it.

As the weeks passed, I held as firmly as I possibly could to that rationale. Every now and then, fear somehow would find its way into my mind and haunt me with visions of going through the whole thing again. After this happened a few times, I developed a pattern for deleting it. I would think of something I had been wanting or needing to do and make up my mind right then and there to do it. This actually served a double purpose. It took my thoughts away from the tumor. And by getting things done, it made up for my tendency to procrastinate at times.

Period of Normalcy

Always a pleasant time of the year, the summer of 1992 came and moved along swiftly. It was not without memory of what had happened one year before, beginning with the telephone call from Dr. Tsaris. What a year it had been since then, but that was behind us now. We were enjoying the summer days and it was better to think of the positive things of today than the negatives of yesterday.

The double vision and facial insensitivity were still with me. Yet, I was reassured nerves can repair themselves, though sometimes it takes years. I hoped mine would be faster. The other aftereffects, aside from a memory still not up to par, had gone.

As to the memory, there was no question it had improved, mainly because my ability to concentrate kept getting better. I had worked hard at it, getting the children to help me so I could help them more with their school work. And I had enlisted Elena to help me with household things I had difficulty in remembering. While I still wasn't back to where I had been before the operation, I was pleased to be rid of the helplessness and frustration I had felt when it seemed my memory had left me entirely.

October came along. A year had passed since the operation. It was time for another MRI. Again I approached the big cylinder with rosary beads in my hand, positive thoughts in my mind. Over the past six months, as before, no symptoms had occurred, no signals had been sent to indicate the tumor had reasserted itself. Furthermore, I had been to Dr. Mazurek for an examination and he had detected nothing to suggest disturbance inside. I was confident everything would be all right.

Dr. Mazurek's telephone call the next day validated my confidence. No growth in the tumor could be discerned in the MRI pictures. Again, a happy outcome.

The days moved into November and time again for Mom to come from Florida to spend Thanksgiving with us. She was thrilled to see how different I was from the year before. We had much to talk about and did lots of things together. As always, it was such a pleasure to have her with me.

We spent Christmas at home. In preparing for it, I succeeded in doing most of the things I had done over the years before the operation. And, believe me, it was a great feeling to be capable of doing them again. Then came New Year's Eve. I thought back to the last one and how I had to pull myself together to enter 1992 with optimism and confidence.

It was with the same optimism and confidence that 1993 was begun. Who could know that before this new year would end, a dark cloud would form and hover over me, a cloud I had hoped never would reappear.

Not Acceptable

Things went well through the first nine months of the year. Richard continued to have to do a great deal of traveling, but did manage to spend a little more time at home with us. The children were doing well in school and were active after school. Susan was a cheerleader and a member of Masquers, the theatrical group at the high school. Michael had taken up lacrosse and already was on his way to becoming a star. Richard II was playing soccer and loving it.

As for me, I was busy with the usual things in connection with the household and the outside activities I always had enjoyed. My vision had not returned to normal. Nor had the feeling on the right side of my face. But I hadn't given up. In April, I had my six-month MRI and there appeared to be no evidence of growth in the tumor.

There was no suspicion that anything would be different in the October MRI six months later. As had been true before, there had been no symptoms or signals to suggest anything had changed. When Dr. Mazurek telephoned the next day, however, it wasn't his usual message that the pictures had shown nothing new. Instead, he made an appointment for me to come to his office to talk with him.

This sounded ominous. I was anxious to find out what the story could be and glad to have an early appointment. What he told me was that in the pictures he thought he had seen some change in the area of the tumor. This might be an indication of some growth or perhaps a shadow from the position of the MRI camera. He suggested we get in touch with Dr. Fraser to discuss it. He was calm and didn't try to alarm me, but thought it important enough to check further.

I became what perhaps only can be described as stubborn. As far as I was concerned, growth in the tumor was not acceptable and I chose to ignore the MRI and what it might mean. After all, I hadn't been experiencing anything that would indicate the tumor had reactivated itself. Why not let sleeping dogs lie? I was sure an MRI picture could be misinterpreted.

It wasn't that I felt Dr. Mazurek was overreacting. I had great respect for him as an individual and as a fine, caring professional who was conscientious in everything he did. It was just that I seemingly had become so strong in my conviction the tumor would remain dormant that I had closed my mind to any other eventuality. This had a definite plus side. It helped me to lead a normal life without worrying about what might be found at some point along the way.

Richard was away at the time and Jeanie was the only person I told about the MRI and Dr. Mazurek's conversation with me. She wasn't sure I was doing the right thing in ignoring his advice; I could tell she was worried about me. When Richard did arrive home, I also told him. He felt the same as Jeanie. But I wouldn't hear of anything other than my own decision to do nothing. I guess I was so adamant in the stand I was taking that both decided it was better not to argue with me about it.

Sudden Happenings

It was around the middle of November, that my long reprieve from pressure by the tumor began coming to an end.

My balance was becoming a bit shaky. I wasn't in danger of falling – not yet, anyway. But I didn't have full control over each step when I walked. Then there was my speech. It was beginning to change. I was speaking at a higher pitch, slurring some of my words, talking faster than I normally did. Obviously the tumor was back at work. Dr. Mazurek had been right. Still, I wasn't willing to give in and do something about it.

Mom came up from Florida for Thanksgiving and she immediately noticed these changes in me. I knew she also was worried and felt I should be getting medical help. But she wasn't one to interfere in our affairs, so she didn't press the point.

We had our usual family Thanksgiving dinner. I felt somewhat embarrassed throughout the day – or perhaps defensive. Here it was, an annual occasion we always loved, all of us together, and my very evident symptoms were putting a damper on the festivity. I knew that all present – Richard, the children, Maryann and Dan, Richard's mother and brother Tony and my mother – were concerned about me and believed I was taking those symptoms too lightly. Why I refused to budge was a mystery to them.

What was in my mind is not hard to pinpoint as I think back to that time. What had begun happening was a horrible jolt to me. I had convinced myself I was in the clear with so much time having elapsed since the 1991 operation. So, it was extremely difficult for me to accept the realization this wasn't true. I know I wondered about things getting worse and whether I was only postponing the inevitable, much as I hated to think of another operation. Certainly I didn't want to think of it. The holiday season was at hand. I recall hoping I could so occupy myself with preparations for Christmas that the symptoms wouldn't matter.

Ironically, those very preparations in mid-December were making it plain that I couldn't ignore the warnings much longer. Negotiating the stairs of our house to hide Christmas packages in my closet suddenly became almost impossible without help. The loss of strength in my legs left no doubt about my deteriorating condition.

Though it wasn't easy at times, I did manage to get through Christmas without major problems. We all knew what would have to be done after the first of the year and there seemed to be a silent understanding not to mar the holiday season with talk about my recurring symptoms.

New Year's Eve. Richard and I sat exactly where we had two years before to say goodbye to 1991 and welcome 1992. I thought about the melancholy mood I had been in as the change in years approached and how I discarded it for a positive frame of mind to enter 1992. And it did turn out to be a good year. Until near its end, so did 1993.

What would 1994 bring? Was my long reprieve over? Would I have to go through the same things again? The steroids, the surgery, the lasting effects so hard to manage. This was the dreaded prospect as the new year approached.

It wasn't a happy outlook as we watched the ball make its 60-second drop at Times Square to signal the end of 1993 and the beginning of 1994. I was scared! I was right back to where I had been the day Dr. Tsaris called to tell me I had a brain tumor. The two words pierced me with the same fear as before. Could I overcome that fear? I decided I *must* and *would* make the effort.

Reflections

Have Follow-up Checks

For whatever period of time a neurologist may deem necessary, it is extremely important to see one on a regular basis after brain surgery. This certainly proved to be true in my case, and I was fortunate to have Dr. Mazurek recommended to me. It was clear from the very first time I went to him that I was in the hands of a thorough professional. He not only would make sure that my tumor was watched carefully, but would do everything he could to help me recover.

Equally important is having a set schedule of follow-up MRI's, or other form of scanning, or other type of checking that may be recommended. By no means is this to imply that all patients have tumor regrowth and other problems such as mine. Rather, it is a matter of being cautious, making certain everything is satisfactory, and if not, finding out what needs to be done.

A mistake I made was not heeding Dr. Mazurek in October of 1993, when he told me my latest MRI indicated some growth may have occurred in the tumor. I was regrettably stubborn about the whole affair. He was patient with me, and as my symptoms grew worse, I had to face up to the fact that he was right. A lesson I learned is that since the objective is to benefit from what the neurologist observes and advises, *it pays to listen*.

Lean on Your Religious Beliefs

Throughout my long experience, my faith kept me from feeling alone. A spiritual presence was always with me. Its being there helped to give me the will and the strength to get through the operations, emergencies, and disappointments, and the perseverance to take me through the long, arduous periods of recovery.

There would be moments when despondency over my impairments would consume me and cause me to wonder whether my faith had failed me and I had been abandoned. But the fact that I could overcome these feelings of despair and could continue on a positive course gave proof to me that I had not been left on my own.

There is no intent here to preach. My own example is offered purely as a suggestion that whatever your religious beliefs may be, before and after surgery are times to hold firmly to it.

7

A Fortunate Lead

An Exploration

Richard played a key role in what unfolded for me early in 1994. No part of my long medical odyssey has been more pivotal than something he did that January.

I didn't know it at the time, but some months before, two close friends of his, Allen Ross and Leon Marrano, had both mentioned to him a story in *Reader's Digest* about the work of a New York neurosurgeon, Dr. Fred Epstein. As I was to learn later, the story told how Dr. Epstein's compassion for children with serious brainstem tumors had led him to make a career of operating on them. The special skills he had developed with tumors at this specific location in the brain had saved many young lives and had contributed significantly to advances in brainstem surgery.

Richard had thought it would be beneficial to talk with this talented doctor who specialized in my type of tumor if it became definite that I would need another operation. Because I seemed to be getting along so well, he had said nothing to me at the time. He hadn't wanted to do anything unless and until it might be necessary and I would agree to it.

At this point there was no question about necessity. My symptoms were getting worse. I was having trouble swallowing, my speech was getting more slurred. Even my vision seemed to be getting worse. Weakness in the left side of my body made it difficult to walk; I was afraid of falling and would have to hang onto things to keep my balance. I had trouble showering for fear of falling, and getting dressed was becoming a problem for me. I felt I was slipping away somehow and losing control of my actions. Everyone could see that something had to be done.

Early in January, Richard told me about the *Reader's Digest* story and how important he felt it was to talk with Dr. Epstein. With so much knowledge of brainstem tumors, his advice would be invaluable to us. Perhaps he would even take me as a patient. I agreed that it would be wise to talk to the doctor, but felt Richard should see him alone for the initial contact.

With the help of Allen Ross, Richard was soon able to get an appointment with Dr. Epstein, and he sent him my latest MRI pictures in advance. The doctor was gracious and cooperative, indeed most helpful. He said he was not the person to do my operation, but emphasized the extreme importance of intimate knowledge that had been gained on dealing specifically with brainstem tumors. He explained why by saying other parts of the brain have backup systems. With them, when one area is injured, another takes over for it. With the brainstem it's different; there is no other area that can take over. In other words, no margin exists for even the slightest mistake.

(We had learned why this is so true. It's because of the density of the nerve fibers there. All these "wires" to and from the brain must pass through this very compact cable. Any injury to a small part of the cable injures many of the wires, and there are no replacements for them.)

Dr. Epstein went on to tell Richard about neurosurgeons who were experts on brainstem tumors in adults. There were five in the world, one in Germany and four in the United States. One of those in this country was in Washington, D. C.

Richard immediately asked him about the specialist in Washington and learned he was Dr. Laligam Sekhar, at the George Washington University Medical Center. Dr. Epstein said Dr. Sekhar was known to have performed more than 100 successful brainstem tumor operations and had an outstanding reputation. He suggested we make an appointment with Dr. Sekhar and send him my latest MRI pictures in advance.

Richard came home highly encouraged and told me about Dr. Sekhar and the fact he had done so many operations on tumors of the brainstem. I agreed that we should see him at the earliest possible time.

Richard moved ahead right away to make the appointment. He had no trouble getting through to Dr. Sekhar on the telephone and giving him a brief rundown on my present condition. Dr. Sekhar said he would be glad to meet with us on February 14th. As Dr. Epstein had suggested, he asked that my latest MRI pictures be sent to him in advance. The appointment was on Valentine's Day – an easy date to remember.

Everything we learned about Dr. Sekhar from a friend in Washington confirmed what Dr. Epstein had said about his outstanding reputation.

A member of the Department of Neurological Surgery at the George Washington University Medical Center, Dr. Sekhar, 43, had his medical training in Madras, India. He did his internship at the Cook County Hospital in Chicago and his residency at the University of Pittsburgh Medical Center. As a neurosurgeon, he had decided at a point in his career to concentrate on brainstem tumors because of the challenge they involved and the shortage of practitioners who centered on them. He had joined the George Washington staff in April of 1993, having gained international attention through the surgical expertise he had demonstrated.

The Interview

Richard and I were both determined to make sure that this time we would find out much more about the operation before it took place, than we had in the past. Such matters as how the surgery would be done, how much of the tumor actually could be removed, what the aftereffects would be.

With these things in mind, Richard asked Dr. Carl Weiss, a Garden City orthopedic surgeon and longtime family friend, to join us for the appointment with Dr. Sekhar. Although Carl wasn't associated with brain surgery in any way, he surely would understand the details as Dr. Sekhar would explain them, and he, in turn, could help us with our understanding. We were very glad he agreed to fly to Washington with us.

We were there at the appointed time on Valentine's Day. I joked with Richard about his arranging it on this date so he could consider the appointment a Valentine gift to me.

We couldn't have been more impressed with the reception we received that day. From the moment we arrived at Dr. Sekhar's office, I had an intuitive feeling that we would be returning.

Dr. Sekhar, a trim man with greying black hair, dark features and eyeglasses that blended with those features, greeted us in a most open and friendly manner. (He spoke to Carl and Richard after his meeting with Richard and me.)

Dr. Sekhar had my MRI pictures on a lighted holder in front of him. He asked me questions about the symptoms I had been experiencing and had me do a few simple tests. One was holding out my hands with the palms up, palms down, first with my eyes open, then with them closed. Next the exercise of following his moving finger with my eyes; also the finger to nose test. Finally he had me walk back and forth to observe my balance.

When these were finished, he pointed to my MRI pictures and said he wanted us to understand from the outset that not all of the tumor could be removed. He explained that the tumor had arisen from the clivus, a part of the skull close to the brainstem, and was compressing this vital cable of nerve fibers. Great care would be needed to avoid endangering those crucial nerves. He did feel, however, that about 75 percent of the tumor could be removed by surgery. This recalled Dr. Lavyne's warning to us back in 1991 not to let anyone try to tell us the entire tumor could be removed. In other words, he confirmed what we already knew.

We assured Dr. Sekhar we had understood this. With 75 percent of it gone, there seemed little likelihood I could have problems from it. We learned from him that a later procedure could reduce its size even more.

He went on to explain that the surgery would have to be in two stages. The first would go behind the external right ear and then through the structures of the inner ear to clear a path to the tumor. Dr. David Schessel, a head and neck surgeon there at the medical center, would collaborate with Dr. Sekhar on this. The operation, a painstaking one to assure minimum disturbance to sensitive brain tissues, probably would take 12 hours. Because it might be necessary to sever a nerve in going this route, I could lose the hearing in the ear.

The second stage would be the actual surgery to remove the bulk of the tumor, much of which would be tough and fibrous. Because of the extreme care needed to protect the nerves of the brainstem, this also would require a considerable amount of time, undoubtedly 12 hours or more.

Dr. Sekhar ended the explanation by saying he really felt he could help me and, if we wished to proceed, he had set aside dates for the two stages of the operation. The first would be on February 28th, the second on March 3rd. We were delighted that he already had decided to do the surgery if asked and, anticipating he would be, had gone ahead to schedule it.

As to aftereffects, he already had mentioned the possibility of losing hearing in my right ear. I could possibly lose the vision in my right eye. While there was no way of telling until he was doing the actual second-stage surgery, there might also be added facial paralysis.

The more we talked, the more my fear of another operation faded. Dr. Sekhar's knowledge of my exact type of tumor and his explanation of the surgery gave me confidence. It was too much to expect that there wouldn't be aftereffects. I had lived with them before and could do it again. The important thing was that I would be rid of the bulk of the tumor. No time was needed to make our decision. Everything about this remarkable surgeon, everything he said told us we were in highly capable hands.

Impressions

Before we left, Dr. Sekhar introduced us to his nurse practitioner, his right-hand person, Margaret Fiore. Margaret, from Brooklyn, was about 5'7" and slender in her white coat. I quickly noticed and admired her reddish-brown hair. After talking with her for a few minutes, I discovered there was much more about her to admire; quickly apparent were her kindness and compassion.

She had great confidence in Dr. Sekhar and he obviously had equal confidence in her. She explained that I always could come to her with questions and that she was available to help me in every way possible. She would be there during the surgery and would be keeping close watch over me during my hospital stay after the operation. All told, I would be there for about four weeks.

Margaret and I have formed a bond of friendship that has lasted to the present time. She was so helpful, understanding, and encouraging that she made my days there as pleasant as any hospital stay can be.

The fact of the matter is we were impressed with everything we saw and heard there on that Valentine's Day. The atmosphere was warm and friendly; it was as if you were regarded as a welcome guest, not a patient to whom admittance was a favor. Particularly comforting was the emphasis on the human touch that was so noticeable, of wanting to go out of the way to be of help.

Our friend Dr. Weiss was greatly impressed by Dr. Sekhar's close knowledge of precisely what had to be done to reach and perform the surgery on my specific tumor. And he was reassured by the doctor's feeling that about 75 percent of the tumor could be removed. So were we. The three of us came home with high respect for Dr. Sekhar as a doctor and as a man.

When we arrived home we found what had been decided in Washington was only one of the good things to happen that Valentine's Day. Michael, a fine student and All-America high school lacrosse player, would be going to college in the fall. He had been interviewed at a number of schools and his preference was Harvard. News had come that he had been accepted. What a joyful ending to the day!

Maryann came over later that evening. Michael had telephoned to give her the good news about Harvard. She wanted to congratulate him in person and was very anxious to hear about our appointment with Dr. Sekhar in Washington. Our enthusiasm in telling her about the doctor, Margaret Fiore, the medical center, and my forthcoming two-stage operation confirmed how pleased we were with what had transpired that day.

It is important to note that we also gave Susan, Michael, and Richard II a full accounting of the Washington visit. We were determined not to repeat past mistakes of holding back from telling them the full story. From their reactions we knew now how much they appreciated knowing what was going on. They were sorry I would be away for so long, but happy that I would be well again. We talked to Lee out in Boulder to tell him too, and he was relieved that our appointment had been such a success.

The children, mentioning that I would be away so long, brought me face to face with that unhappy reality. Four weeks would be quite a while to be away from home. How would everybody get along?

Getting Ready

Richard, on the other hand, was worried about my being alone for much of the four weeks I was in the hospital. He said he would try to arrange things at the office so he could spend some time in Washington beyond the weekends. I hadn't really thought about being more than 200 miles from home for the long stay.

It soon developed that others had thought of the same thing; we had no need for worry about my being lonely. Maryann and Dan told us they already were making plans to be on hand a number of days. And Jeanie was working things out to be with me as often as possible.

It soon became clear that I wouldn't have to worry about things at home. As they had done in 1991, Maryann and Dan were planning to come over evenings to be with Elena and the children when Richard was away. And the fact Elena still couldn't drive a car would be no problem. Carolyn Casano and Nora Forelli said they would see to it that one or the other took her wherever she needed to go. And they would take care of after-school driving, as would Fran Carlson, the mother of Susan's best friend.

Since everyone knew I was going through difficulties with effects from the resurgent tumor, it was plain I was being relieved of having to think about responsibilities. This was a great plus for me. With my mind at ease about the children, I would be in a much better state mentally to handle the operation.

The warning Dr. Sekhar had given me that I might lose hearing in my right ear was something that did keep entering my mind, however. It wasn't that I was any less determined to accept it and live with it if need be; rather, it was a case of being more than a little intrigued by the first stage of the operation – going through my inner ear to clear a path to the tumor.

When Maryann and I had explored the brain and brain tumors in the library before the 1991 operation, the research had embedded in me a desire to have more than superficial knowledge about the medical aspects of my case. My conclusion at that time was that having such information was of benefit to the patient in understanding the *why* of medical decisions.

It was time to go back to the library. I fully trusted the strategy Dr. Sekhar had decided on in clearing a route to the tumor. But it just might be that the medical encyclopedia would help me to visualize the route for myself and to understand the logic of using it. My attitude already was positive; this would add confirmation to why it should be.

When I asked Maryann whether she would join me in the return expedition to the library, of course she was enthusiastic. Her point of view was that no patient could have too much medical knowledge about his/her own case, and she was glad to have the opportunity of helping me with my search.

I also felt it was only fair to let Dr. Mazurek know what was going on. He certainly had been right in wanting me to find out about another operation, and I felt he was entitled to know where this stood. He appreciated this, wished me success in Washington, and asked me to let him know how everything worked out.

A Return Visit

The medical encyclopedia was right where it had been before and just as imposing as we remembered it.

We both recalled how impressed we had been with the illustrations showing intricacies of the brain. We had the same reaction now as we studied the ear. I was astounded at how little I knew about the fascinating structure of the organ that enables us to hear. Maryann was more familiar with it, but we agreed that it's so easy to take for granted vital organs of our bodies and not bother to find out much about them until something goes wrong.

We looked at the first of two illustrations portraying in color the anatomy of the ear. This showed the visible part of the organ – the outer ear – and the one-inch canal leading from it to the eardrum and a small cavity known as the middle ear. The second depicted the inner ear, a labyrinth of winding passages and canals deep within the bones of the skull. By turning the pages back to the section on the brain, we could tell approximately where this was with relation to the tumor on the brainstem below. What readily became apparent to us was the logic of taking this route to the tumor. The canal from the outer ear provided an already existing passage into the brain through sensitive tissues and nerves.

Much as this existing pathway might facilitate getting to the tumor, one thing was clear. This would not lessen the need for the most skilled of surgery. We had the utmost confidence this was precisely what the surgery would be on February 28th and March 3rd. Maryann and I were proud of ourselves for what we now knew about the magical process by which we hear.

The February days went by. Richard and I would be leaving for Washington on Wednesday the 23rd and I was anxious to get there. I felt my control of things was ebbing constantly. It even had become almost impossible to sleep; I kept feeling I was going to fall out of bed. The operation couldn't be over too soon as far as I was concerned.

I had been watching the Winter Olympics on television. I decided that the operation would be Dr. Sekhar's and my personal Olympics and we would win the gold. There will be more on this later.

Reflections

Being Informed

A point was made earlier about the desirability and advantage of learning as much as possible about the brain, the tumor that has grown inside, and the operation that will be done.

What Maryann and I had seen and read on our former visit to the library was of great help in understanding Dr. Sekhar's explanation of the two stages of the operation. This understanding was enhanced by our return visit to the library to study the ear and the route that would be traveled to get to the tumor.

Knowing how carefully the tumor's type and location had been analyzed in determining and planning the required surgery was of real help to me in building confidence in the outcome. Some patients may not want to know so many details in advance; that, of course, is a matter of personal preference. Based on my own experience, I recommend finding out all about the tumor operation, the expected aftereffects, and the follow-up needs.

For Family and Friends

There always was so much to do on a day and night schedule that I worried about how Elena and the children would handle things. What a relief it was to find out that all these concerns were taken care of by my family and friends.

8

The Resumed Journey

Under Way

If we had believed weather could be an omen of what was ahead, we would have been discouraged about driving to Washington that Wednesday, February 23rd. Richard had worked things out to be able to stay there through the second phase of the operation on March 3rd. He would need his car, however, for trips into Maryland and Virginia in connection with his work. Jeanie had arranged to go with us to help with anything I might need the first few days of my stay. We had planned to leave around 10:00 A.M. for what would be a drive of five or six hours. Of all days to get up and look out at the start of a major snow storm!

The flakes were beginning to come down in gusts and the radio forecast was that the storm would continue for several hours as far south as Baltimore. We debated about starting out under such circumstances. Knowing I was scheduled for preliminary tests the following day, Richard felt we should go ahead and leave as soon as possible. His reasoning was that we would be on main highways all the way and could get through before enough snow might accumulate to close them.

It wasn't a drive I would ever want to repeat. The snow came down so heavily at times that it was almost impossible to see out of the car. The whole thing was pretty scary to Jeanie and me, but though he frequently had to grope his way along, Richard didn't let it stop us. We did arrive in Washington late that afternoon and went to the hotel where we had rooms reserved close to the medical center. Jeanie and I had been nervous coming through the storm, but the snow had stopped and thanks to Richard we were safely there.

The two tests I was to have were scheduled for Thursday afternoon. We had the morning free, and spent it touring the Georgetown area of the city. This was our first visit to Georgetown with its beautiful town houses and other sights. We enjoyed every minute we were there.

I checked in at the hospital early in the afternoon. Two tests were scheduled. First was an audio examination and measurement of my hearing ability. A machine called an audiometer was used to produce electronic sounds of different intensities and frequencies. The machine made a graph showing the range of my hearing. It seemed likely, perhaps almost certain, that the forthcoming surgery would cause me to lose hearing in my right ear. This made it important to assess the capability I would have with the other ear. I was assured it would be good; the left ear was in excellent shape.

The second examination was an EEG. It's no wonder they use the abbreviation for this 20-letter word: electroencephalogram. (It was spelled out at my request to know what the initials meant.)

In this test, several small electrodes were attached to my scalp. These led from an instrument I was told would measure and record all sorts of impulses in my brain. The recording procedure lasted about 45 minutes. Impulses were measured under a number of different circumstances. These included with eyes open, then closed; while and after breathing heavily; while looking at a flashing light; and when thinking hard, then just letting the mind relax. From what I could understand, the purpose was to assess the different nerves in my brain and their capacity to bounce back from the long hours of anesthesia and disturbance they would undergo in the two stages of the operation. Obviously, they passed the test.

This night was one of my last two outside of the hospital walls for some time, and Jeanie, Richard, and I "lived it up" at a restaurant recommended to Richard. We splurged and had the best steaks topped off with big ice cream sundaes.

More Preparations

Friday it was back to the hospital for two more tests, observations and consultations, a new MRI, and to stay overnight.

The first test, an angiogram (blood-vessel images), was not pleasant because of what seemed like endless time lying perfectly still on my back, experiencing hot and cold sensations. Dye had been injected into one of the arteries supplying blood to my brain and this flowed to the vessels inside. When enough dye had circulated in the vessels to give them clear contrast, a machine took X-ray pictures. These, highlighting the vessels, would serve two purposes. They paved the way for a follow-up embolization I was to have. And they would provide Drs. Schessel and Sekhar with added guides for the delicate, precise surgery they would be doing.

When I was told an embolization would be next, I had to know just what it was; somehow the word was foreboding. The explanation given to me by Dr. William Bank, who would perform it, was that it involved the deliberate blockage of blood vessels. In some cases, this was done to stop internal bleeding. In others such as my case it was to cut off blood supply to the tumor.

Through the same artery that carried the dye to my brain in the preceding angiography, a thread-thin flexible tube (catheter) was guided by television monitoring (flouroscopy) up into the major blood vessel supplying the tumor. Through this tube a blood-clotting agent was deposited to close the vessel.

These procedures, which were so routine to the professionals who carried them out, were completely amazing to me. We read and hear about the great advances medical science has made, but until we have firsthand experience with them, we can't be fully aware of how miraculous some of them are. The more you learn about them along the way, the more confidence you have as a patient that the right things are being done.

That evening I was taken to another area for something that had become quite familiar to me over the past three years – an MRI. Dr. Sekhar wanted it in order to compare the post-embolization pictures with those from my last MRI.

The main reason for keeping me in NCCU (Neuro Concentrated Care Unit) overnight was to observe how well I had withstood the series of tests and procedures. Whether it was from going through so many of them or from a reaction to being in the hospital for the first night, what little sleep I had was fitful. I understood the importance and necessity of these tests, but undergoing them had been an ordeal that worried me. Would I be able to take in stride the two long, critical operations that were ahead? I knew this was no time to let fear creep back into my mind, but it was difficult to keep from being apprehensive. I was released at 10:00 that Saturday morning to return on Sunday.

Jeanie, Richard, and I decided that I needed a complete change of scenery. Off we drove to Baltimore. Richard had told us about the wonderful development some years back that had transformed the city's Inner Harbor into a showplace.

The three of us had such a good time. Views, activities, shops, eateries and other attractions make the

Inner Harbor a popular mecca for residents and visitors alike. For a late lunch, we had Baltimore's famous crab cakes. For me, the afternoon was a welcome respite from the hospital procedures of the past two days.

By the time we got back to our hotel, I was in much better spirits. In contrast to the night before, I had no trouble falling asleep and had a restful night.

Stage One

My return to the hospital was set for late morning on Sunday. Richard was up early and ate breakfast before Jeanie and I had showered and dressed. The two of us decided we didn't want to bother with a real breakfast and joked about the nutritious value of what we had as a substitute – diet coke and chocolate bars with almonds.

Jeanie and Richard took me to the hospital at the scheduled time and checked me into my assigned room. They stayed on, we watched television, and so the hours passed.

In mid-afternoon a handsome young doctor came in. He explained that he would be inserting a "central line" into my chest. I understood that this was a pre-cautionary measure that would provide direct access to my blood stream for blood samples to be removed or medicine administered.

This would be done in the morning. He wanted me to know about it so I wouldn't be surprised, and maybe upset, at not having been told. I wasn't looking forward to this procedure, having the tube implanted in my chest, but I did understand the importance of his telling me about it.

A bit later Dr. Schessel came in. We were pleased to meet and talk with him. Since he and his team would be performing the first stage of the operation, he wanted to be sure we understood just what it would involve. He referred to it as mastoid-type surgery on the right ear to remove the mastoid bone and part of the inner ear. With a dead space then exposed, there would be an open approach to the tumor. He was sorry that the result could be loss of hearing in that ear, but the essential task of removing as much of the tumor as possible made this risk necessary.

My research with Maryann made it easy to understand Dr. Schessel's explanation. I didn't tell him we had done this, but did say I was fully aware of the possible loss of hearing in the right ear. I thanked him for coming in and told him I was confident in what he and Dr. Sekhar would do.

Jeanie and Richard left around dinner time. Monday would be a big day with an early start. They felt I should have a quiet evening to myself. It didn't end, however, without a visit from Margaret Fiore, Dr. Sekhar's nurse-practitioner. As noted earlier, Richard and I met her during our first visit to the medical center. She had a relaxed way about her that gave me both confidence and calmness. What an invaluable friend she has become.

Good friends Anne and Len Bullock had come to Washington from their home in Charlotte. Len appeared with Richard at the hospital at 6:30 A.M. as I was being taken to the pre-operation area. It was a comfort to know they would be with Richard through-out what would be a long day. Jeanie had arranged to visit some friends in Arlington outside of Washington.

Richard was allowed to go with me to the pre-op area where I was for a short time just before being wheeled into the operating room. The surgery took about 10 hours. Richard had called Margaret Fiore to find out how I was doing and she arranged for him to meet with Dr. Sekhar at around 5:00 P.M. The doctor told him everything had gone well and was in place for the second stage of the operation.

It wasn't until 7:30 P.M. that Richard was permitted to come to the recovery room to see me. He wrote in my diary that my head was covered with bandages and my face was so swollen I couldn't talk, but I was alert and could squeeze his hand in answer to questions. Also I was extremely thirsty, but only could have very few ice chips to melt in my mouth. He made a notation that the thought of my having to go through so much made him feel cold and clammy, but he realized there was no choice.

Later that evening I was taken to the intensive care unit (ICU) where I spent the night. All I wanted was to fall asleep and not think about anything. Thanks to sedation, this was what happened. The next morning, Tuesday, I was moved back to my room.

Tuesday and Wednesday went by slowly. The swelling in my face gradually lessened and I was able to talk in a hoarse whisper. Jeanie visited me during the day, Richard came in the evenings. Television helped pass the time, and I would doze off occasionally. I remember small pleasures like the ice cream Richard brought me Wednesday evening, the night before the big day of stage two.

It was fortunate that I was able to sleep soundly that night and not think about what was in prospect. Had I had any inkling of what was in store for me following the second stage of the operation, the night would have been a devastatingly long one with no sleep whatsoever. I had every confidence in Dr. Sekhar's skill and faith in my ability to survive. But I had no premonition of how extensive and tenacious the after-effects would be.

Stage Two

It was another early start that Thursday morning, March 3rd. I was wide awake when Richard arrived at 5:00 A.M. with Jack Wehrum, a dear friend from Garden City. Jack was in town for the day and wanted to be sure he saw me to wish me luck. How thoughtful friends can be.

Jack left in a few minutes to let Richard have time with me alone. Dr. Sekhar and the anesthesiologist who would be attending me arrived to chat briefly with us before I was taken to the pre-op area. I suggested to Dr. Sekhar that as long as he was doing all this, he might as well give me a face lift. But, as the four of us laughed about it, I added that since he would only be working on the right side of my face, it might look peculiar. I also mentioned to him that I looked upon the operation as our personal Olympics and we would go for the gold. He squeezed my hand in assurance we indeed would do that.

Richard told me later that the anesthesiologist said I reminded him of Tom Wolfe's book, *The Right Stuff*, about the first American astronauts. I've thought of that many times since when I've needed to reassure myself that I would overcome lingering obstacles.

Another friend, Neil Donovan, had come from Philadelphia to spend the day with Richard. Though they stayed busy, Richard put in a number of calls to Margaret Fiore. Twelve hours after the surgery had begun, she told him Dr. Sekhar was finishing and would meet him in ICU.

They met at 7:15 P.M. The good news was that Dr. Sekhar had succeeded in getting about 80 percent of the tumor. He felt the remaining part of it could be controlled by Gamma Knife radiation. This could be at a later date.

Successful as the operation had been, however, there were more adverse side effects than we had expected.

It had been impossible to avoid severing a nerve that could mean permanent loss of hearing in my right ear. We had come to accept this as a definite possibility, so it came as no surprise. The right side of my face had additional numbness, but this could subside eventually. We also had anticipated this.

On the other hand, learning that I would have weakness on the left side of my body for some time and would have to use a walker to keep from falling came as a shock. So did the prospect of having to be fed through a tube (PEG) into my stomach because my swallowing had been affected. This had been inserted immediately after the operation while I was still sedated and I was not fully aware of its purpose until later. Not only that, but one of my vocal cords was injured and I was unable to talk. Moreover, I might have to have a tube in my windpipe to assure getting sufficient oxygen to my lungs.

A plus was that I hadn't lost the sight in my right eye. But, because of the numbness in that side of my face, the eye had no feeling. A brush of my hand or a speck of dust could cause infection or damage to the cornea without my being aware of it. So the eye had to be sewn shut temporarily to prevent any possible harm.

There was no question about my being happy with Dr. Sekhar's having removed so much of the tumor. But at the same time, there was no way I could keep from being stunned by so many things that I had had no idea would happen to me. Could I adjust to them? I wasn't sure. My positive thinking had been pierced and I was at an all-time low.

During the long night, when worries and fears can become magnified into visions even worse than the realities, I wasn't even sure I wanted to live with so many things wrong with me. It wasn't that I *thought* I would die; it was that I almost *wished* I would. Never before had such a thought even remotely entered my mind. Now that it had, it was not to be the last time.

Rough Days

The next day, Friday, I was still in ICU. Doctors maintaining a continuous check on me were concerned about my breathing. Margaret Fiore told me it had been decided that I would have a procedure called a tracheostomy. This would involve making an opening in my windpipe (trachea) and inserting a tube to provide a clear airway for oxygen to get to my lungs. Dr. William Wilson, chief of the Division of Otolaryngology (head and neck disorders), set this up for Wednesday when I would have gained some strength.

Meanwhile, a temporary tube in my mouth served the purpose. It was a terrible annoyance and led to an incident that caused a great deal of commotion on Saturday.

By now, I was back in my regular room. Richard had brought his walkman and some country music he knew I liked. As we listened, the tube began bothering me, so as a natural reaction I pulled it out. Richard was scared to death and rushed out to get help. After 10 minutes of confusion, the tube was back in and I knew I would have to force myself to resist pulling it out again.

I remember Sunday as a terribly unhappy day. I was agitated about that tube in my mouth, and depressed about not being able to talk or walk or eat normally. On top of all that, the side of my face was numb. It was also weak, and there appeared to be danger that it might droop. I was horrified with the thought; how would I look to the children? How could I go anywhere without being ashamed of my face?

The only way I could communicate was by writing notes – terribly unhappy notes – and Richard was the unfortunate person who had to bear the brunt of them. My frustration had reached a point of not only filling me with anger, but making me confused and irrational. I would write notes asking the same questions over and over. Why am I like this? Why have these things happened to me? Have I had a stroke? I must have had a stroke because my face will droop. Where will they take me? What's to become of me? Why are they keeping me alive? Why don't they let me die?

Richard was great. He was unbelievably patient and reassuring. I had had no stroke, he kept on telling me. My face wouldn't droop. I would look just the same as I always had. All these things that had happened were only temporary. By no means would they ever let me die.

On Monday afternoon I did have the tracheostomy to insert an airway tube into my windpipe. At the same time, to protect my injured vocal cord and to help it to recover, a small piece of plastic (thyroplasty) was set in next to it, serving as a form of bandage. This could be removed easily, but I was urged to let it stay there to aid the healing process.

Richard was diplomatic in telling me later how I reacted to just about everything during those days immediately following the operation's second stage. Cautious as he was in what he said, it was plain my temperament had been far from exemplary for a patient. He did go so far as to say I seemed angry with everyone and everything. And he was right. My mind was consumed with the negative things that had happened. I was so angry and feeling so sorry for myself that there was no room for being rational about the all-important positive: Dr. Sekhar's success in removing so much of the tumor. This kind of thinking was out of character for me, but I guess not too surprising under the circumstances.

A frightening thing that happened that Tuesday compounded the situation. I had managed to quiet down somewhat from being so upset and depressed. Lying in bed sort of dozing, I began hearing a thunderous noise. It was as if a giant machine were moving closer and closer to me, with the terrible noise it was emitting getting louder and louder. I covered my ears as if it were noise from outside, but that of course was futile. The noise was inside my brain and so frightening I thought for sure it would be my undoing. Then it stopped.

Jeanie, who had become alarmed by my description of this strange sensation, ran out into the hall to find a nurse or doctor. The doctor she found explained that the sensation of loud noise could be from pressure on the brain from swelling or fluid. This, an aftermath of the operation, would subside in time. It did after a few more episodes over the next several days. I dreaded the noise itself and the awful feeling my brain would explode from it.

Making Progress

The rest of the week went by slowly. Late one afternoon. I was sleeping when a commotion of sorts wakened me. The floor nurse was trying to find out who my gentleman visitor was. In what seemed like seconds he placed a small package on my hospital table and disappeared. Although I couldn't actually see his face, I knew instinctively who he was. Richard arrived a short time later and unwrapped the package. Inside was a small pair of lovely crystal rosary beads. He wanted to know who had left them. We played a sort of game, with Richard asking questions to which I could only shake my head yes or no. Within minutes he knew my visitor had been Joe Carabetta, a longtime friend from Connecticut. How thoughtful it had been of Joe to take the time to come and to leave such a precious gift.

Saturday I had another delightful surprise. Anne Keating came down from New York to visit me. It was great to see her. Also Richard returned from a short trip he had to make. He telephoned the children and Elena from my room to report my progress. They knew I couldn't talk, but it was wonderful to hear their voices. They told me how much they missed me and were looking forward to my being home. That, however, would not be for a while.

Sunday was a banner day. With a little coaxing from Anne and Richard, two nurses washed my hair.

What a marvelous feeling! My spirits improved. I began to think about recovering from the depressing effects such extensive surgery had created.

Monday morning, March 14th, a milestone was reached. I was able to sit up in a chair! Jeanie was so excited when she arrived and saw me that she made me feel as if a major celebration were in order. For that matter, I guess it was. Every step forward, however slight, was worthy of being considered an accomplishment.

That same morning I met three therapists who would be working with me the next two weeks. This was the beginning of a new learning experience about three types of rehabilitative work that have become large and extremely important components of modern medical science.

One of the professionals, Maria, would be my physical therapist, concentrating on my walking, balance and strength. Because of the weakness on my left side, my leg, knee, and foot nerves and muscles needed certain exercises in order to regain strength and rehabilitate themselves.

Linda was to be my occupational therapist, working to restore fine motor skills such as hand movement and coordination that had been affected by agitation to nerves in my brain.

Susan Fantom, speech pathologist at the medical center, was the third therapist. She would be helping me with my throat by working with me to overcome my swallowing problem and to get my voice back. Our association continued after I left the hospital. As with

Margaret Fiore, she has remained a friend I can call on when I need advice.

It was at this point that I was moved to 6 South, the rehabilitation floor. Every patient's name was listed on a large white board near the nurses' station. Beside each name was the time the three therapies – physical, occupational and speech – were scheduled for the day.

All the therapists were wonderfully skilled in the ways they guided and helped us to go from what often seemed utter helplessness to being able to do essential things. There can be real frustration in feeling you should be capable of doing things you can't do. Over time you come to understand that each part of the therapy is designed to play a role in bringing back the capability. That's why you're there.

Speech was hardest for me. Along with the swallowing difficulty and inability to talk, I couldn't move my mouth properly. Try as I might, I couldn't even smile with both sides of my mouth. Susan Fantom was always encouraging, though. She kept telling me that although I couldn't speak or eat then, the day would come when I would look back on all of it as just a bad memory.

Happy Sides

Speaking of memory, there were incidents and occasions that bring smiles when I look back to my stay on the rehabilitation floor.

How well I recall when I could bathe myself in bed without help from the nurses. They were delighted with my progress in being able to do it, and one of them – we called her by her initials, B. J. – crowned me "Queen of the Bed Baths."

That wasn't the only title I was given. Louis Cappelli, a close friend of Richard's, sent me two gorgeous bouquets of light pink roses over a period of a few days. They made my room so fragrant that some of the nurses took to calling me "The Flower Lady."

Then there was the business about the bathroom. When they finally let me begin going there, a nurse would always go in with me. This seemed to have a delaying effect on my being able to do what I was in there to do. This caused one of the nurses to say to me, "You must have a bashful bladder. I'll get out of here. You ring me when you're ready." I could pull a cord to give the sign I was ready, and that became the procedure for humoring my "bashful bladder." (It worked!)

How patient nurses have to be in such matters! And what admiration and respect you develop for them in being the recipient of their dedicated understanding and compassionate care.

Often I think of one of them, Susan, who had an obsession about moist lips. She thought every patient should have them and would check to make sure before letting us be taken to other floors. "You can't leave the room with dry, cracked lips," she would say. "What would the other floors think? Let me take a look at you."

A tape our son Lee had sent us from Boulder provided some amusing and entertaining interludes. Lee's talent for music had led him to join a small band at the university. On the tape was a song they had written, "Walk Like a Chicken." It really was a very catchy tune, and I enjoyed listening to it. So did others. Every time I played it an orderly or one of the transportation persons, who took patients in wheelchairs to different therapy rooms, would come in and put on little dances. When they found out it was our son's band, I became very popular.

The days passed. Soon I was dressing myself, putting on a wig and a touch of make-up and I had my first "field trip." We were three patients, each in a wheelchair accompanied by our therapists. We went to a little doughnut shop about two and a half blocks from the hospital. There was a fresh, invigorating feeling of spring in the air, and I thought about it as the season of rebirth. For me, that's what it was – a rebirth of faith and confidence, putting behind me the despair and anger that had gripped me after the operation.

The therapist who was with me hadn't realized I was being fed through a tube and couldn't have anything in the doughnut shop. She apologized and took me on a window-shopping tour around the small commercial area while the others had coffee and doughnuts. It was fun being out, a thrill just to breathe that lovely air.

An Escape

Jeanie, who had spent so much time with me, had to get back to Long Island to catch up on her work. I insisted she go. After all, she had been so faithful that I couldn't possibly ask or expect her to do more for me in Washington.

Meanwhile, Maryann and Dan arrived on Saturday, the 19th. Dan was to return home late Sunday afternoon, but Maryann would stay on for several days. It was a treat for me to see both of them and I was so glad Maryann could stay. They reassured me everything was going well with the children, Elena, and the house. I couldn't help worrying about being away so long and was pleased to have these first hand reports that everything was all right.

Sunday was a beautiful day and the four of us – Richard was there – thought we should take advantage of it. Like four criminals, we planned the perfect crime. We would "break out" and tour the city.

With the excuse we were going to the cafeteria, we launched our escape. Richard went to bring the get-away car to the exit we decided would be the best one to use. Maryann was the lookout. Dan's job was to look as nonchalant as possible as he wheeled me right out of the hospital and to the waiting car.

We were proud of ourselves as we drove around the city, laughing like school kids getting away with some unbelievable prank. Buds were appearing on the trees in Washington's beautiful parks and we talked about how pretty the city would look in April. We stayed out as long as we dared, enjoying the "freedom," then went back to the hospital in time for my next feeding. What a happy interlude it was. A really exhilarating experience for me. I was so glad we did it and began to think of it as my personal version of "The Great Escape."

When Dan left a short time after we returned, he took with him a note I wrote to the children telling them how much I was looking forward to being home with them soon. This was Maryann's idea. My handwriting had improved so noticeably over what it had been before the operation that she thought the children would be heartened to see it.

Dan also left a suggestion with us that proved to be of great help to me. At night I would get scared and frustrated when I couldn't communicate with the nurses' station. I would press the button by my bed, the light would go on over the door of my room, I would hear a voice over the intercom asking what I wanted, but since I couldn't talk, I couldn't answer. They would think my ringing was a mistake and there I would lie unable to do anything about it. The whole thing was scary. What if I were choking? What if something were wrong with me?

Dan said the thing for me to do was to have my wheelchair right next to the bed during the night. I could shift over into it by only getting my feet to the floor. This would be no problem for me. My balance was still affected, but I could stand on my legs. In the wheelchair, then, I could wheel myself out into the hall and to the nurses' station.

Maryann and Richard told the chief night nurse about this plan, and she agreed that it would be a good idea. From then on, the wheelchair was close beside me, and nights became much less worrisome to me. We were glad that Dan had come up with this easy solution.

Busy Days

Good ideas run in the Daly family. Maryann had another one. Susan Fantom had given me mouth and throat exercises to do in my room. I seemed to have more difficulty doing them than I should have, so Maryann worked out a game to help me. I would try to smile, she would grimace. It got to be a very funny ritual. After a while, she even added sound effects. Anyone walking past the room had to wonder what we were up to. But it all worked. Susan commented on my progress.

Something else Maryann did was to help me with things I couldn't remember. It sometimes seemed my short-term memory had been lost entirely. I couldn't recall things shortly after they happened. I was assured I would regain it over a period of time, but it was a serious handicap to me for a while. To make up for it, Maryann put my clothes out for me every night so I would know the next morning what I had decided to wear; I now could dress myself. She also would write on a board across from my bed what day and date the next day would be. And she got me a clock to keep in sight so I could be sure of the time.

Richard was able to stay in Washington for a few more days and Maryann and he were permitted to take me out for short trips around the block or to a small park across from the hospital. With the large scar on the side of my head, I got my share of stares in the wheel-chair. Richard, always an economist, thought it would be a good thing for me to hold a tin cup in my hand; he reasoned that, after all, every little bit of income would help. I laughed along with him and Maryann about this "clever" idea, but after that I never let them talk me into going without my wig.

The days were full. There were visitors from Garden City and other places where we had friends. One, Bob Silverman from Atlanta, brought me something I'll always treasure – a small, blue glass bird, a gift from his wife Carol. It was, Bob explained, the bluebird of happiness which was to watch over me until my recovery.

Something that impressed me as being ironic was the fact a dining room was directly across from my room. I could watch the patients eating and smell the food and think about how real food would taste. But I had to accept the tube as a fact of life – at least for the time being. That food did smell good, though!

If I had any tendency at any point then to feel sorry for myself about something, seeing a young woman whose room was near mine quickly dispelled it. She had had a stroke, and it showed in what had been an attractive young face. Her two children, one boy three years old, the other five, would come to visit her and I wondered about their reactions to her condition. She would be going home soon and I hoped so strongly – and prayed also – that strength and normal appearance would return to her.

Friday, March 25th was an especially happy day. Lee was on his way home for his semester break and made a detour to come to see me. Again, there was an "escape." Lee wheeled me out of the hospital to a spot where Maryann and Richard were waiting in the car. Off we drove to Annapolis. What an enjoyable lark it was and especially wonderful being with Lee. He said he was relieved by the way I looked and acted, but I wondered. I was really afraid that I would scare the other children.

The Big Day

April 1st was set as the date I was to leave the hospital. Maryann arranged to stay in Washington until then. Richard had to go back to Garden City, but would return to drive us home. I began counting the days.

Once home, I would have to continue with therapy. The hospital wanted to be sure adequate facilities were available in or close to Garden City, and Gary Gregory, senior social worker at George Washington University Medical Center, did a good deal of telephoning to check. He gave us the information he obtained and it was up to me then to make a choice. The main thing was to proceed with it as soon as I could after arriving home.

Two days before we were to leave, Susan Fantom took me downstairs for a test called a video swallow. This impressive technique had been developed to examine one's swallowing capability by X-ray photographing of the throat as small quantities of liquids of different consistencies are tried. A camera positioned near one side of the head takes the pictures and these are shown on a screen at the other side. The test showed that I was still aspirating – the liquid was going into my lungs instead of my stomach so I would have to continue being fed through the tube, but Susan and Dr. Sekhar assured me that eventually the swallow would come back to normal.

As for the tube, Maryann and Richard were becoming experts in feeding me through it with the liquefied nutrients that comprised my daily diet. An occasional mishap resulted in a lap full of liquid, but this was happening less and less frequently. Soon the skill would be passed on to Elena. She would have to carry on until the happy day I would be able to eat as a normal human being.

Susan and Dr. Sekhar also left no doubt that my voice gradually would come back. Every once in a while I could utter a throaty sound. This was an indication the injured vocal cord was healing.

Preparations for home started on Thursday. It had been a long hospital stay and I wanted to be back where I belonged. As much as I was looking forward to being home, I would never forget the kindness of the many wonderful individuals who had helped me.

April 1st arrived. Good Friday. Margaret Fiore came to my room in the morning to make sure everything was ready for my release from the hospital and to say goodbye. I would miss her, but knew I would see her again; there would be return visits to the hospital. A little later, I was being wheeled to the car. It was a lovely day. The air felt fresh and invigorating, quite a contrast from the snowy February day five weeks before.

A season had ended, another had begun during those five weeks. For me, another segment of my long medical journey had been traveled and a new one was ahead. There would be more hills to climb, more turns to make. With Good Friday as the starting day, how could I have anything but a confident outlook about climbing those hills and negotiating those turns?

Reflections

The Deep Sleep

As I reflect on my two hospital experiences, I keep thinking about something that is probably not a common observation in offering advice to patients. It has to do with the oblivion one enters and stays in while the surgeon is doing his work.

To consider how many hours I had been "out" in the sense of being totally unaware of what was going on – even feeling nothing when a knife was cutting into my brain – is to realize how crucially important the anesthesiologist is to the surgeon and to the patient. Here again, it is essential to have confidence in the professional responsible for administering exactly the correct dosage throughout the entire operation, regardless of how long that may be.

The key to that confidence is talking with the anesthesiologist beforehand. In each instance, the one who would be with me came to the pre-op area to tell me what would be done and to answer any questions I might have. The result was that in my mind there was no doubt whatsoever that I would have excellent vigilance. My recommendation to any patient who will be given anesthesia is to welcome and take advantage of the opportunity to talk with this critical practitioner.

Being Considerate with Nurses

One of the wonderful nurses at George Washington University Medical Center said something interesting to me about relations with patients. There is a fine line, she said, between giving the patient needed help and being invasive. Doing the right thing depends on knowing when to retreat and let the patient be alone. How true this is. There are times when there is need for something to be done or someone to talk with, there are times when privacy is what will help.

On the other side of this coin is a fine line it is up to patients to observe. There are times when nurses are so busy they can carry out only the most essential of their duties. There are other times they can stop to visit or do other little things that haven't needed urgent attention. Unless this situation is an emergency requiring quick action, it is only fair for the patient to be conscious of the timing factor. If you have given that consideration, nurses can be your best friends during a hospital stay.

A Tip for Visitors

It was my own experience – and other patients have said the same thing – that sometimes improvement can be so slow it's hard to keep from being frustrated and angry. Other observers are usually in a better position to judge improvement than the patient who is so close to the day-to-day situation. Whenever even the slightest gain becomes noticeable, encouragement is ignited by telling the patient so and elaborating on its significance.

This is true not only in the hospital, but also after going home to recover. Being assured of progress is *very* therapeutic.

9

Capital Improvements

Happy Reunion

What a thrill it was to be home. Lee had returned to school in Boulder but I was so excited about seeing Susan, Michael, Richard II, and Elena that my "condition" temporarily was put out of my mind. My heart was filled with the joy of being with them; nothing else mattered right then.

On the drive from Washington, I hadn't been able to escape having some apprehension about how they would react to my arriving home possibly needing a wheelchair, definitely needing a walker, being fed through a tube in my stomach, partially deaf in one ear, with a strange-looking closed eye, and not being able to talk. But thanks to Dan, they had been well prepared on what to expect.

During the early part of my hospital stay, he and Maryann had gone out of their way to spend time with the three children at home, keeping their spirits bolstered and reassuring them I would come through the operation successfully. Later, when Maryann was with me at the hospital, Dan had been perfectly frank with them about the aftereffects, telling them it would take time for me to be myself again, but with their help, I would succeed.

So all three tried hard to conceal the shock and sadness they might really have felt in seeing me. They told me how wonderful it was to have me home, how much they had missed me, how they and Elena and their friends had prayed for me every night. They were enthusiastic and upbeat, but I could detect some lip-biting to hold back surging emotion as they looked at me and faced the full reality of my "handicaps." My awareness of this made it difficult to keep from crying, but they were being brave and it was up to me to display the same strength.

Over the Easter weekend there were many heartening telephone calls, to say nothing of beautiful plants and bouquets of spring flowers. I was somewhat overwhelmed by all that had been and was being done to make my homecoming such a major event. Again, as had been demonstrated in so many ways, I knew that no one could have been more blessed than I was to have such a loving family and so many warm, devoted friends.

Monday morning I reminded myself that it was time to get on with recovery. Gary Gregory knew I would have to continue with therapy after I came home and had made all the necessary preliminary arrangements. I would be going three times a week to the rehabilitation center at the office of our friend Dr. Carl Weiss in Garden City. From the time he had gone with us to Washington to talk with Dr. Sekhar, Carl had been in contact with us to make sure everything was going all right and to offer his help in every way possible.

As she had been all along, Jeanie again was there to help. She arranged her schedule so she could drive me three times a week to and from Carl's office. This wasn't easy. It meant getting me from the walker into the car, folding the walker and putting it in the trunk, reversing the process when we got there, then doing the same thing all over again to get back home. Jeanie was quite adept at it, though, and so cheerful about the whole thing that she kept me in good spirits.

At the rehabilitation center, I met my therapist, Pat. Her first objective was to evaluate my situation. She designed a program which involved a series of exercises to strengthen my legs, knees, and hips. She was very considerate in bearing with me; therapists have to have infinite patience. This was especially true in my case because I could not communicate very effectively. But we did move ahead and Pat had me begin my sessions with a ride on the stationary bicycle, followed by a series of weight lifting exercises, and then a workout involving either a peg board or large rubber bouncing ball.

It soon became apparent to Pat that I was favoring one side of my neck. My right side had become "stiff." When I turned to look to the right, I was moving my whole upper body instead of just my head. She made a recommendation that became a part of therapy I began

looking forward to – massage. Pat would begin by
manipulating the right side of my neck from the base of
my jaw down to my shoulder. Slowly she stretched the
muscles to allow more mobility, a sensation that was
both slightly painful and wonderfully soothing.

Mom arrived from Florida on April 11th. She had
said she would come to help whenever the best time
would be, and this seemed to be it. Who could know
everything would come to an abrupt halt two days later?

A totally unexpected development resulted in an
emergency trip.

Back to Washington

Mom noticed something when she was cleaning
the incision in my neck that had been made for the
tracheostomy. Tiny bubbles were oozing from it. She
was concerned about infection and felt we should call a
doctor right away. We quickly put in a call to Margaret
Fiore, feeling they should know about it at Dr. Sekhar's
office. Margaret, obviously concerned, wanted to know
whether I could get to Washington that day or early the
next day. This was impossible so she asked me to be
there as soon as I could. Meanwhile, I was to get to the
closest available neurosurgeon and have him examine
the troublesome area. We were able to make an appointment with Dr. David Chalif in nearby New Hyde Park
and Mom drove me there the next morning. Dr. Chalif
examined my neck, took a small sample for laboratory
analysis, and showed us how to clean the area to avoid
infection.

Richard was out of town on business, so the next day Jeanie came with me again to Washington while Mom took care of things at home. When we arrived in Washington, I checked into the hospital and waited for what I assumed would be a series of tests. I was right; the tests began at once. It was now April 15th.

The tracheostomy incision was swabbed and again a sample taken for analysis. The next step was to check the shunt that had been put in after my first operation at New York Hospital and had to be moved slightly during the surgery in Washington.

A small hollow needle about 1/2" long was used to extract some fluid from the shunt. Because this was on the side of my head that had no feeling, there was not the slightest sensation of pain. It took a few days before Dr. Sekhar felt confident that the bubbling was not due to infection. Though the cause seemed to be a mystery, we were more than relieved that the drainage had been controlled and we had nothing to worry about.

While I was there, a decision was made to remove the stitches and open the right eye that had been sewn shut to prevent infection and corneal abrasion. This proved to be excruciatingly difficult. The upper and lower eyelids had begun to fuse. This necessitated potentially damaging work to separate the two.

The resident doctor performed this task at a painstakingly slow pace. Sometime later I looked into a mirror and was horrified at what I saw. From being in one position for so long, the muscles in my right eye had atrophied. The eye held left of center and couldn't move to the right at all. My immediate reaction was to call Margaret Fiore. She in turn called Dr. William Geist, the medical center ophthalmologist, who had sewn the eyelids together.

Once again, an injection of botulinum toxin was productive. Although I was not able to move my eye all the way to the right, I could move it about halfway. There was absolutely no feeling in it, though. The nerve that had been traumatized in the 1991 operation had not yet repaired itself but I had the hope it would at some point.

By the time Jeanie and I had arrived back from Washington, Richard had returned. Everyone was surprised to see how different I looked with my eye no longer sewn shut. I still had double vision, but at least my face had a closer resemblance to the old me.

Now it was back to therapy, with Mom driving me. She stayed until the end of April. She was so patient about feeding me through the tube and helping me in countless other ways that the first month would have been much harder if she hadn't been there.

Day by Day

As slow as it was, physical progress was steady. I was using the walker most of the time, but hadn't entirely abandoned the wheelchair. It was nice to use it for sitting out in the yard to enjoy the spring sunshine and fresh air. We were always going to spend more time out there, but somehow spring, summer, and fall went by without our getting to it. Schedules were too busy to permit much time for that sort of thing. Now, as I sat there absorbed by the beauty around me, I thought of how much we had been missing. It was time to do some rearranging of schedules.

Before Mom left for home, one more happy event occurred, and she and Elena were the first other persons to witness it. I was able to speak in a hoarse whisper. It happened in the kitchen. Mom and I were about to leave to go shopping and we had made a list. It was on the counter near where Elena was standing and I automatically tried to say "grocery list." All three of us heard the whispered utterance of those two words. If I had been capable of dancing, I would have, and the other two would have joined me. We were sure my voice was in the early stages of returning.

This might mean also that my ability to swallow and eat real food was started on the road back. What a celebration there would be when that day came! Often I would think of things I would eat first, but it was impossible to make up my mind because there were so many foods at the top of the list.

My whispered "grocery list" was but another in a series of accomplishments, however small, that could be equated to climbing Mt. Everest. Taking the first shower after the operation. Washing my hair by myself for the first time after requiring a nurse's help. Taking the first step out of a wheelchair and into a walker.

Standing for the first time and keeping my balance without holding onto something. Each of these "little" things meant another measure of freedom regained.

A lesson I have learned from the therapists who have helped me is to be willing to adjust, to do things in a different way, but to do them. There are obstacles to rise above. The secret is to persist in finding new ways to make the climb.

The Face in the Mirror

There was another aspect of therapy that was in its way just as important as the physical exercises. There is a natural feminine desire to look good, even for one's own family. Scars from the surgery didn't make it easy to do and I was never without my wig. With great encouragement from my friend and hairdresser, Ben Paulino, I was able to face the world without hiding under that wig.

The hair on the side of my head that had been shaved for surgery had grown in coarse and gray. Ben recommended we color it back to its natural shade. Having done this, he went to work shaping my hair into the most attractive style. I was apprehensive about having short hair for the first time in my life, but I was thrilled with the results. His expertise was solidified by the rave reviews I got from friends and family alike. No psychotherapist could ever have given me a more positive boost than Ben was able to do with those magic scissors.

The Mental Side

There was no question about my physical progress from the therapy program, but I was in a frustrating struggle with a combination of other effects. This was something I had to work out on my own.

Problems I had after the first operation – short attention span, memory lapses, loss of confidence – had persisted for some time. Gradually, though, by taking the time to concentrate hard on what others were saying, on remembering even little things, and on forcing myself to make decisions, I was able to improve. I hadn't come back 100 percent, however; there were times I still had memory difficulties.

Now, the lingering effects from unavoidable disturbances to the brain were different.

One extremely strange problem was my inability to walk through a store in a normal way without getting a violent headache that would require the person I was with to take me home where I would have to go to bed. I just couldn't look at so many counters and displays at the same time. What I had to do to prevent the painful phenomenon was walk with my head down looking only at the floor until we would reach the area we wanted.

The same thing would happen when I was riding in a car and would try to look out the window in a normal way. I couldn't look at so many things at once. The motion of the car made it worse; I took to keeping my eyes closed and resting my head on a pillow to lessen the motion.

The reason for the violent pain, it seems, was that some of the nerve fibers controlling my eye movements and balance had been injured in the operation. They would come back eventually, but meanwhile caused pain when called on to perform such complex tasks as viewing many objects at the same time. It took some weeks for healing to take place; what a relief when I finally could walk through a store and look around, or ride in a car and be able to look out the window.

Another pronounced effect caused me to regret my reaction at times. Things that never bothered me before would trigger quick agitation. I would magnify little incidents into big irritations and flare up over them. Because I could speak only in whispers, I was limited in the angry words I could utter, but my gestures would leave no doubt about how I felt. I had always been able to keep my temper in check, but now I seemed to have no control over it. It had to be unpleasant to be around me during these episodes, and I know they were especially hard on the children. Aware of this, I would resolve to stay calm and rational, but something amiss in my brain would bring a repetition of the uncalled-for flare-ups.

To their credit, the children and my friends were understanding. They did everything they possibly could to be patient with me, knowing I wasn't myself and hoping I would be soon. I hoped and prayed for the strength and discipline to restore my self-control and lead me to act as a sensible, rational human being.

As with so many other things, it was a matter of time. I had been told the brain would heal itself from the minor injuries to its nerves. It was healing that had to take place in order for me to regain full control of my ability to reason, to use good judgment, and to make proper decisions. I wished the recovery would come faster, but the important thing is that it did gradually come.

Something quite unusual happened June 1st. I was sitting with Richard II watching television when I began to cough. I coughed and coughed so violently that I could hardly catch my breath. Frightened at my behavior, he ran to get Elena. She helped me up, hoping that walking around would help. Then I coughed up a small piece of white plastic. By chance, Maryann stopped in just as all this was taking place. She immediately called Dr. Sekhar's office and explained what had happened. It sounded to him as if I had coughed up the thyroplasty, the small plastic device that had been inserted to hold my vocal cord in place until it healed. This was not considered an emergency, but since I was scheduled to be in Washington a short time later, I was advised to make an appointment with Dr. William Wilson, who had inserted it.

Achievements

In therapy, one learns to be thankful for every little bit of added capability and improvement. Each advance, however slight, is cause for celebration.

My progress was wonderfully satisfying to all of us. Early in May I had been able to take what to me was a giant stride, moving from the walker to a four-pronged cane. Things went so well with this prop that by the end of the month, I could walk confidently and safely with just a regular cane. A marvelous feeling of achievement came with each of these steps forward – from wheelchair to walker to four-pronged cane to ordinary cane. Next would be the accomplishment of them all – the ability to stand and walk entirely on my own. I visualized how rewarding it would be to have that freedom again.

June 26th was Michael's graduation day from Garden City High School. Mom had come back north to be there for it and to spend more time with me. Most of the family would be at the graduation exercises in the school stadium. I walked with my cane to our seats in the stands. When the ceremonies opened with singing the "Star Spangled Banner," I rose with the others and stood with no difficulty. My cane was leaning on the seat where I had put it.

My thoughts took me back to the day I left the hospital in Washington. I had shared my private goal with Margaret Fiore. My goal to be standing, unassisted, at Michael's high school graduation. I made it!

July 13th was another date not to be forgotten. An event of immense importance and meaning to me took place that day at the hospital in Washington.

From the time speech pathologist Susan Fantom had begun working with me to bring back my ability to swallow and to talk, I had been doing throat exercises. Recovery of speech had progressed now from hoarse whispers to hoarse words. The muscles that control swallowing had been slow in healing, however, necessitating my being fed through a tube all the months since my operation. With mid-July having arrived, it was time for my third video-swallow test. I was extremely anxious, even nervous, about it because I wanted so much to be able to eat normally.

Maryann flew with me to Washington. When she had been there and had spent so much time with me at the hospital, she had become acquainted with Susan Fantom and the video swallow. It was a great plus to have her along. Having fed me so many times through the tube, always telling me the day would come when I no longer would need it, she was as anxious about the test as I was.

Susan sat me in what had become a familiar straight-back chair with an X-ray camera at shoulder height on one side and a screen on the other. I watched her mix powdered barium with water. Teaspoons of this would tell the story. She had explained to me before that barium is a metallic chemical impervious to X-rays. This makes it possible for the camera to show images on a screen of how the substance is being swallowed and where it goes.

As Susan reached toward me with the first teaspoon of the barium mixture, I felt my body tremble from the tenseness of knowing how much was riding on what would go on inside my throat in the next few moments. All eyes were fixed on the screen. We could see the throat muscles moving. The barium was going down . . . . . yes, into the correct tract, going to the stomach, none into the airway to the lungs. A "safe swallow" was clearly visible on the screen. Could it be true? Another teaspoon, the barium swallowed slowly, the same safe trip down. And another the same. It was true. The magic day had come.

But that was only the first half of the good news for the day. My appointment with Dr. Wilson was to find that I had indeed coughed up the small one-half-inch piece of plastic called a thyroplasty. Dr. Wilson was quite amazed. He had heard of this happening, but never to one of his patients. This was a first for him. Maryann and I teased and told him we thought he should have it bronzed.

The conclusion was that my having coughed up the little protector was a sign my vocal cord was healing well and no longer needed it. For my voice began improving noticeably from that point on. So, this was another day for celebration.

On the plane back, Maryann and I made a list of things I gradually could begin eating. Jello would be first, then ice cream and puddings. From these I could branch out to soft bread and pasta. The "permissibles" would widen after that and I was looking forward to all of them.

The following weeks were interesting. When I was able to keep expanding the menu, Maryann experimented with all sorts of things. It was so enjoyable just to know I could begin trying to eat normally. This happened gradually, however. The liquid tube feedings were still my main source of nourishment, with "real" food gradually being introduced.

Eating was not the same as it had been before. Every swallow had to be done slowly and carefully after chewing each bite and really concentrating on what I was doing. I ate all my meals alone. No conversation could be included. My throat could not handle doing both things together, for fear of choking.

Late in August, through a cautious course of progression, I was able to eat just about everything. August 27th became another memorable date. Thin liquids were the last items to be authorized, and on that date I had my favorite beverage – my first diet cola since February. On the same day I drove a car for the first time in 1994.

It was still necessary for me to have some of my nourishment through the feeding tube, however. This continued until October 5th. It was then that I had an appointment at the Long Island Medical and Gastroenterology Associates in Great Neck. I was surprised at how quickly and easily Dr. Jay Merker removed the tube. I was happy to have it out, but realized that the device had served a life-sustaining purpose for many months.

A New Adventure

After the operation, Dr. Sekhar had mentioned the possibility of my having Gamma Knife radiation as a means of reducing the tumor still further. He explained at the time that about as much of it as was possible had been removed by surgery. The Gamma Knife would take over from where it had been necessary to leave off. He deferred making a definite recommendation until he could study results of an MRI six months after the operation. That meant toward the end of August.

That time had come. As he had before, Dr. Mazurek arranged for the MRI to be done in Rockville Centre. As with every other time, I went with my wooden rosary beads for a session inside the now-familiar cylinder. I had no fear whatever that anything negative would show in the pictures. There had been absolutely no hints of tumor activity in my brain and I was positive everything would be favorable.

Dr. Mazurek was pleased with the pictures; nothing new appeared to have happened. He sent them on to Washington and in a few days we had a call from Dr. Sekhar. He said he would like to talk with us, that he definitely felt now I should proceed with the Gamma Knife – and he made an appointment for us to see him.

The Gamma Knife. An intriguing name for precise radiation. We were soon to find out much more about it. Another mile in the long medical journey was about to be traveled.

Reflections

Do Your Therapy

Before coming face to face with the need for it, I had little idea of what was involved in therapy to restore muscular action and coordination lost in body muscles through disruption, or injury, to brain nerves that direct and control them. Once I began having therapy, as frustrating as it was at times, I developed an appreciation of how logical it was. Every single exercise had a specific purpose. And I found the people who conduct it to be highly dedicated and qualified technicians.

For patients about to have it, I have two pieces of advice. One, ask the therapist about the purpose of each exercise. Knowing the specific reason for it increases the incentive for doing it. Two, have a regular schedule and keep to it. It's wise to resist the temptation to put it off because it may interfere with something else you'd rather do.

Keep on Looking Your Best

It's amazing how meaningful attention to personal appearance can be in aiding progress with recovery from negative effects of surgery. To have the feeling of being fresh and attractive looking is to have higher spirits and greater confidence in going forward.

As brought out in this chapter, what my hairdresser did for me was therapy just as important as the physical exercises. Frivolous as it may seem, an enthusiastic "you look great today" is an excellent recovery motivator. And a comment I must add is that it's not applicable only to women patients and what might be attributed only to feminine vanity. Male patients with whom I have spoken say the better they think they look the more self-confident they are about their progress.

Family members and friends can play pivotal roles in this form of therapy by being especially observant. It's surprising how much every little compliment means.

To Family and Friends

Another way family and friends can help is not to push the patient to do things until he/she is ready for them. It took a long time for me to feel up to going to parties. I loved socializing with two or three friends at a time, but for reasons I can't explain, I didn't want to be in larger groups. I know other patients who have had similar experiences.

Since there are likely to be qualms of one kind or another as a natural aftermath of serious brain surgery, helping the patient to overcome them gradually is the preferable, more beneficial course to follow.

10

The Invisible Blade

Precision System

The meeting Richard and I had with Dr. Sekhar was encouraging. We recalled our first appointment back in February and all that had happened since then. He was pleased with my recovery and still held hope, as I did, that I would get over the double vision and that sensation would come back to the numb side of my face.

In telling us about the Gamma Knife, he described it as "radiosurgery" – a system that forms a concentrated blade of radiation beams produced by radioactive decay of cobalt 60. These beams penetrate the tissues in precisely targeted areas of the tumor. As they do so, a process of cell destruction is created within the tissues. In the majority of cases, this results in actual death of the cells. Shrinkage in the tumor observed in follow-up MRIs confirms the death. But since cells in a tumor such as mine are slow to grow, they can also be slow to die. So MRIs may be necessary for an extended period of time.

Dr. Sekhar said we would learn more later about just how the technique works; the important thing now was to make arrangements for proceeding with this further step. He assured us I would be perfectly safe in all respects; the only harm would come to the tumor.

Richard and I both had so much confidence in Dr. Sekhar that we had no hesitation about going ahead with Gamma Knife treatment.

After meeting with Dr. Sekhar, we looked in on Margaret Fiore. As always, it was good to see Margaret. She had followed my progress, giving me encouragement all along on the telephone and on my trips back to the hospital. She was enthusiastic about my having the Gamma Knife treatment and said Dr. Steiner, who would be doing it, had a great track record; I would be in excellent hands.

While at the hospital, I also visited with Susan Fantom. Only a few weeks before she, Maryann, and I had danced for joy over my video swallow test showing that my throat muscles were strong enough for me to begin eating a few foods. She was interested to hear how many different things I tested and tasted since then. And she commented on how natural my voice was beginning to sound. With one deaf ear, it was harder for me to judge the sound of my voice, but I did feel it was getting better and was pleased to get her professional opinion.

All in all, this was a fulfilling visit. I suppose it's a bit strange to be nostalgic about a place where I certainly had my share of depressing, rough times, physically and mentally. But it wasn't too hard to block these from my mind and think of the positives: the accomplishments in therapy and the encouragement I received on the rehabilitation floor.

Moreover, in no way could I overlook or forget the fact I had gone to the medical center with a dangerous tumor causing me all kinds of distress and fear. Weeks later I had returned home with aftereffects, yes, but more important, with a priceless gift.

I had been released from the grip of a growth inside my brain that could have ended my life after drawn-out suffering.

Impressive Record

We arranged for an appointment with Dr. Ladislau Steiner, Director of the Lars Leksell Center for Gamma Knife Radiosurgery at the University of Virginia Health Sciences Center in Charlottesville, on September 1st. Richard went with me, of course, and we arrived at Dr. Steiner's office anxious for a favorable response. The more we had considered Dr. Sekhar's positive feeling about the Gamma Knife, the more convinced we were that my having the radiosurgery was the logical and smart thing to do.

Dr. Steiner's manner immediately made us comfortable. He was a man of medium build in what we guessed to be his late 60s, wearing green operating clothes and walking with a cane. He spoke with quite an accent; he was born in Romania. He and Dr. Sekhar were colleagues at the University of Pittsburgh. In

Sweden, he had collaborated with the late Lars Leksell in development of the Gamma Knife. His center at the University of Virginia was one of 20 such sites that since had been established in the United States. Two qualities that quickly inspired confidence in him were his own self-confidence and self-assurance.

Something else that came through clearly was his very cautious approach. He wanted to be absolutely sure the Gamma Knife was right for the particular case being considered. After participating in developing the technique, he had performed his first operation with it in Sweden 18 years before. Since then he had done more than 2000 of the operations, half of them on brain tumors. But over the same period of time, he also had rejected a large number of cases because he felt the Gamma Knife was not the answer for them.

Dr. Sekhar had said to us that in my case the Gamma Knife would serve as a second step to the surgery he had performed. Dr. Steiner explained this further. He said brain tumors might continue to grow if residual tissue is left after normal surgery, as had been necessary with mine. If Gamma Knife is used to treat the residual, the rate of recurrence can be cut drastically. He went on to say that he never had lost a patient from Gamma Knife radiation. The way he said this and the expression on his face told us the results he had achieved had been very satisfying to him.

Dr. Sekhar had given us a good idea of how radiosurgery works and Dr. Steiner gave us interesting background information on it. He told us how Lars

Leksell, a gifted young neurosurgeon, was convinced that something new was needed in neurosurgical techniques. He envisioned reaching into the brain with a narrow beam of some kind; in his own words, "I was born under the sign of the 'archer' and looked forward to sharpshoot into the brain." The result of his pursuing this goal was the first Gamma Knife which treated its first case in October of 1967. Because of the technique's successful record over the years since, its use for brain tumor surgery has consistently increased as new centers have been established to make it available.

In talking about the Gamma Knife's benefits, one of the things Dr. Steiner mentioned made me particularly happy. There would be no hair loss or scars. The explanation for this was that the radiation dose is received only at the points where the beams converge to pierce the precise tumor areas inside the skull. This protects against hair loss, scars, and disfigurements often linked to conventional radiation.

After we had talked a while in his office, Dr. Steiner took us down the hall to view the object known as the Gamma Knife. What we saw was a striking piece of equipment – a sleek high-tech "couch" with a large red dome at the end. I was entranced with the entrance to the dome, an artfully shaped aperture one's imagination easily could transform into an entranceway to a magical globe. I could envision myself lying there absorbing the magic.

Seeing the whole magnificent machine put me in an imaginative mood, and that was good. Everything about the visit was encouraging.

We also were shown the helmet I would have on my head inside the dome. This amazing device I'll describe later was part of the whole dramatic instrument medical science and technology had produced to create the miraculous treatment called radiosurgery.

On our way back to Dr. Steiner's office, we met his wife, who is also a doctor. As we chatted with her, it was plain she had as much faith in the Gamma Knife as her husband. She hoped I would be back for the treatment and assured us it would be both painless and effective.

Sitting in Dr. Steiner's office again, Richard and I looked at each other. There really was no doubt in our minds about going ahead and we asked him about a date. He said I could be admitted Monday, September 12th, for treatment the following day, which was fine with us. The sooner the better!

Coming Adventure

Fully assured the Gamma knife was the right thing for me, Richard and I returned home to explain to our children and friends all that we knew about this process.

Gamma was easily explained; it was pretty generally known the word had to do with radiation. But knife? It had an ominous sound. How did radiation and a knife fit together? Fortunately at Dr. Steiner's office Richard and I had looked at a brochure from the company that manufactures the equipment, where the Gamma Knife was referred to as "the invisible blade." This impressed us as being a perfect description for the confluence of radiation beams that penetrate precise targets of tissue. And it certainly served our purpose well in providing simple explanations for the treatment I soon was to have.

The more persons we did tell about the machine and the process, the more an aura of adventure arose around my forthcoming treatment. It was as if I were going on an expedition into a different world and would have much to reveal when I came back to this one. No one appeared to have the slightest question about its being a successful trip. Nor had I. My outlook remained positive.

The few days until September 12th went by rapidly. Before we knew it, we were on our way back to Charlottesville and my "wondrous adventure." With time to spare, we went on a tour of the University of Virginia campus. This led us to recall from our childhood history what we learned about Thomas Jefferson.

From Monticello, his fascinating home overlooking the city, he used a telescope and survey instruments to lay out this campus, considered to be one of the most beautiful in America. He is said to have been a great admirer of the Renaissance style of a 16th Century Italian architect, Andrea Palladio, and the buildings, though they have a colonial appearance, actually are known as Palladian. The entire campus is a magnificent monument to this brilliant, versatile man who left so much that has endured through all generations since his time. It is no wonder thousands of visitors to Monticello every year are enthralled by examples of his genius for invention.

Standing in front of the campus chapel, I thought of something a friend who was a graduate of the university told me. She and other girls she knew had loved this chapel so much that they wanted to come back there to be married when that time came. A surprising number, including my friend, had done just that.

When we went inside, we could understand why there would be such feeling. We were so taken with it that we remained for a while, the two of us sitting there in silence. It was a setting for quiet meditation, for thoughts of belief, of prayers, and of faith.

Reverie took me back to my own prayers from the time of that fateful Friday afternoon telephone call from Dr. Tsaris late in June of 1991. They were pleas for courage, determination, and strength in facing and dealing with whatever might confront me regarding the tumor. These continued through the operation at New York Hospital. Even in days and nights of discouragement over the lingering aftereffects from toxins in my body, there were rebounds knowing patience and efforts were sure to bring answers to my appeals.

During the long reprieve from the tumor's pressure on my brain I had slipped. I didn't stop praying by any means; that never had happened from the time I began as a child. But when I had made up my mind the tumor would stay inactive, there didn't seem to be need for continuing to ask for help with it.

That changed of course when the tumor reasserted itself and we had the good fortune to find out about and meet Dr. Sekhar. In again asking for the kind of help I needed and had been given at the time of the first operation, I added two promises. One, when concern about the tumor was behind me, life would be taken less for granted. The expression "take time to stop and smell the roses" may have worn thin over the years. But no words could have applied more aptly to what I intended to do. The other promise was *to write a book telling of my experiences* in hopes that it could help others facing a similar situation. These were promises I repeated as Richard and I knelt for a few moments before leaving the serenity of that lovely chapel.

Learning More

At the appointed hour of 3:45 P.M., we arrived at the hospital and I checked into a fabulous room with all the latest comforts. There couldn't have been a nicer way to begin my Gamma Knife adventure than to be assigned to such luxury!

The nurse, Doris, came in a few minutes after I got settled and took my vitals. They were all fine and she told us that other staff persons would come in during the evening. Dinner was served early, usually the case in hospitals, and Richard went off for his.

Dr. Steiner's nurse-coordinator Clare came in shortly after dinner and told us what the schedule would be for the next day which would begin at 5:00 A.M. Being wakened at that hour wouldn't bother me; fortunately, I've always been one to get up early!

The next visitor was Dr. Dheerendra Prasad who had come from India to study under Dr. Steiner. A man in his early 30s, of medium build, and with tortoise-shell glasses rimming his dark eyes, he was high in his praise of Dr. Steiner and the Gamma Knife. He and Richard carried on quite a conversation about neuro-surgeons and their specialties and about the role of the invisible blade.

Dr. Prasad impressed us as being a dedicated, bright young neurosurgeon. He said there should be a good deal of serious dialogue between doctor and patient, that what is technically correct as a general rule is not necessarily correct for everyone. He pointed out that Dr. Steiner had turned away patients he didn't truly believe he could help, and at the same time, had helped patients whom others had written off – all of which emphasized the importance of being with the right doctor.

He mentioned something extremely interesting about this. He predicted that advances in computer net-working of information through such systems as Internet would enable individuals to seek out doctors who are right for their *specific* problems. We hear much about the exciting new era of information computers have opened globally. It well may be that Dr. Prasad's forecast is a preview of what is in the future for selecting doctors.

We moved from that conversation to his telling us some technical things about the Gamma Knife, praising Dr. Steiner highly for his role in its development and for the outstanding record he has compiled in using the technique to benefit patients. What Dr. Prasad had to say added to our already-strong confidence in Dr. Steiner and the Gamma Knife.

Our next visitor was Father Justin Cunningham, a Dominican priest. A pleasant coincidence quickly came to light. He was from Jersey City, but after becoming a priest, was stationed at St. Mary's in New Haven, Connecticut. Richard had grown up in Hamden, the next town in Connecticut, and I had gone to college in New Haven. St. Mary's was well known to both of us. So, we had much in common to talk about during the half hour Father Justin spent with us. He also had great admiration for Dr. Steiner and gave us further assurance the treatment would be successful.

It was then that one of the nurses came in and told me it was time for me to take a shower and wash my hair with an anti-bacterial shampoo she brought with her. I would have to repeat both of them in the morning. The reason, she explained, was to provide a sterile skin environment for the helmet that would have to be attached to my head in four places.

At 9:00 P.M., another preparatory step was taken. A plastic tube (cannula) was inserted into one of the veins in my arm to serve later as the entry site for infusion of intravenous fluid. This would be started in the morning to prevent dehydration. I would have nothing to eat or drink until the Gamma Knife treatment was completed.

By this time, Monday-night football was on – the Chicago Bears vs. the Philadelphia Eagles. Long ago I had switched from being a weekend widow during football season and had joined Richard at the television set. I had become almost as much of a fan myself, so it was no surprise that we watched the game to the end. A good and typical way for us to spend this particular evening. Richard left for his hotel after that and I tried to settle down to get some sleep; 5:00 A.M. wasn't many hours away.

Getting Started

When she came into the room those few hours later, my next nurse, Tina, didn't have to waken me. I'm sure I wasn't the only patient who, anticipating the day ahead, had slept very little if at all.

As I had learned the evening before, my having another shower and hair shampoo was the first action in getting the big day under way. The second, around 5:30 A.M., was starting the intravenous fluid.

It was about half an hour later that Dr. Prasad arrived to take me to the pre-op area where there were several different waiting stations. He was so cheerful and made me feel so relaxed about what was ahead that he had me smiling. And I was delighted when he put me in station 12. Since 12 is my lucky number, this made me happy about the way things were going.

Dr. Prasad said he had to leave to do some things, but would be back for me in a little while. It was about 7:00 A.M. when he returned and took me to an operating room. Dr. Steiner was there waiting for me. Two nurses were there also and a visiting doctor, Robert Slawson from Baltimore, who, as an observer, would be on hand for the entire procedure.

The nurses helped me to get onto an operating table. It was completely raised at one end and I sat with my back against it, straight up. A helmet-like steel frame was placed on my head. Its purpose was to enable MRI imaging to establish precise locations on the tumor for the concentrated radiation beams to attack. It was to be attached securely to my head with screws. I would be given local anesthesia for this procedure, one shot on each side of the forehead, two in the back of my head.

One of the hospital nurses had told me that each of these shots would feel like a bee sting. When I mentioned this to the nurse who had come into the room to give me the shots, she must have wanted to prepare me for the worst.

"That's right," she said. "A sting from a bee the size of a 727 airplane. But it's over quickly."

That really set me up. Actually, it turned out to be more like getting four shots of Novocaine from the dentist. Although it wasn't pleasant, I guess I was pretty stoic about the whole thing. And this prompted a comment from Dr. Slawson:

"You women are the ones who hold up well in situations of this kind. The big, burly men are the ones who pass right out."

He chuckled at my explanation. "That's why women are the ones who have the babies."

After that, two of Dr. Steiner's Gamma Knife nurse assistants, Clare and Marion, took me to another room where they put a Lucite dome over the frame. They used this in some way to measure different areas of my head and mark numbers on a checklist. Then they took me to a room that had an object very familiar to me – an MRI machine.

The Lucite dome had been removed, but the frame was still on my head when I was set to be moved inside the MRI cylinder. There was a special cradle for the frame as I lay on my back, and plenty of support was put under my neck to make me comfortable. Marks on the frame would show in the pictures about to come from the MRI imaging. These would be used to help pinpoint the Gamma Knife targets.

In I went. I had had so many MRIs that they had become easy for me. This one seemed to go well and when it was finished, I was taken back to my hospital room to wait for the next activity. The frame was still on my head and another nurse, named Judy, stayed to be sure I was all right. Richard also arrived. He had brought his camera with him to take some pictures of the Gamma Knife. Our telling about the machine had aroused so much interest at home that we thought everyone would like to see photos of it in color. Dr. Prasad had told us this was the only red Gamma Knife machine in existence. It had been built to Dr. Steiner's exact specifications and he was glad to have us take some pictures back with us.

While we waited for the next procedure, I had quite a crisis. I reached under the blanket for my wooden rosary beads. They weren't there. My hand searched frantically; I could feel them nowhere. I had them with me in the MRI cylinder; never did I have an MRI without them. What could have happened to them? I was getting almost panicky. But Clare saved the day. She found them tangled in the sheets on the side of the gurney that had transported me from the MRI to another area before I was returned to my room. What a relief when Clare, a happy smile on her face, held them up to show them to me.

The Main Event

In about 45 minutes, with Richard accompanying us, I was taken to the Gamma Knife area. Dr. Steiner and Dr. Prasad were studying information in computers in front of a large window facing the Gamma Knife room. Everything known about my tumor was in these computers to aid in arriving at a precise plan for directing the Gamma Knife's radiation beams. It was fascinating to hear that two chairs for watching the computers were the original ones used with the first Gamma Knife in Sweden. Dr. Steiner had purchased them and had them shipped to the center when he established it at the University of Virginia.

At 1:00 P.M. everything was ready and I was taken into the Gamma Knife room. Richard came in with us to take the pictures of the machine. The frame was still on my head and I asked Dr. Steiner whether I could take it home with me as a souvenir and conversation piece. He showed his sense of humor by smiling, looking admiringly at the frame and saying he just couldn't bear to part with such an old and trusted friend. But the metal friend and I could be a photogenic duo, he thought. Along with pictures of the machine, why not have Richard take some of me wearing the headpiece? Richard readily did so.

Back to the Gamma Knife, it was a bit of a shock, and certainly a surprise, to learn the procedure about to begin would take two hours or so. I hadn't realized it would be that long, but the reason for it quickly became clear. Six separate areas of the tumor had been selected as targets through combined MRI imaging, computer processing of information, the measurements of my head marked on the frame, and analysis by Dr. Steiner and his associates. Each of these six areas – they're called isocenters or shots – would be radiated separately. So, there would be six individual treatments, each lasting about 15 minutes.

When I got onto the machine's hydraulic couch, I was asked to lie flat on my back. A large helmet, a technological marvel containing 201 portals (collimators) for focusing the radiation beams, was attached to the headframe I was still wearing. With my head thus propped up, towels were placed to support my neck and shoulders. Dr. Steiner told me not to panic when my head was inside the dome. With one word from me, I could be out of the machine in seconds. I would be able to see out into the room and was sure there would be no cause for panic.

Now I was ready to go. My head was moved inside the magical red dome. There were no bright lights, there was no pain or other sensation. Dr. Steiner played classical music, and it was soothing. (I was told some patients even sleep !)

After 15 minutes, I was slid out and a slight change was made in the position of my head. Then back into the dome. This occurred six times in order for the radiation to be directed to each of the six target areas of the tumor. I wasn't conscious of anything going on inside my brain, however, nor was there any sound from the machine. The Gamma Knife's blade not only is invisible, but does its penetrating without the patient's feeling it.

One thing, though, it gets hot inside the red dome. By the end of the six treatments, I was cooked. So I was glad when they sat me up and unscrewed the heavy frame that had been on my head for a long time. This didn't hurt, but it was a strange sensation to have my head free again. Dr. Steiner wrapped my head in a bandage to prevent bleeding from the four areas where the helmet had been attached.

Back in my room, I was tired and hungry, not having had anything to eat since the night before. There were no side effects from the treatments, although a slight pain did develop in the back of my head where one of the screws had been. Medication helped with this.

Richard went down to the cafeteria to get me anything to eat! He came back with a tuna sandwich, a diet cola, and some cookies. Only problem was the cookies were too small. The Gamma Knife did nothing to my appetite, obviously!

Then we called home. Susan answered and we gave her several names to call to say everything was all right. We were both falling asleep after this long, long day.

No lying awake that night! I slept right through until a beeping sound wakened me around 5:00 A.M. At first I was puzzled, but then discovered it was the intravenous fluid device signalling that a new container of fluid was needed. This was taken care of promptly by one of the nurses. I tried to get back to sleep, but once awake, I was too excited about going home later in the morning.

Dr. Steiner arrived at about 7:30 A.M. He was wearing a suit and tie, and this was the first time I had seen him without medical clothes. He wanted to know how I was and I told him I felt great. He examined the bandage on my head and removed it with one quick pull. I asked him about the outcome of the Gamma Knife treatments. Although he told me nothing definite, his answer did give me confidence the radiation had been successful.

"We'll have to wait six months for an MRI to tell us," he said. "But from our knowledge of your tumor and the areas we treated, I think the results will be positive. We must wait to know for sure, however. Meanwhile, please enjoy living a normal, happy life with your fine husband and family."

His sincerity came through so genuinely that I couldn't have been more grateful that we had connected with this great doctor. I thanked him and told him how very much we appreciated what he had done.

At 8:00 A.M., the nurse came back to remove the intravenous fluid device. Now I could take a shower and feel more like myself again. Richard arrived soon after, and Dr. Prasad and Clare and Marion came to say goodbye and wish me well. The interest and regard all three had shown for me as a person, not just a patient, were heartwarming. Dedicated as they were to their professions, they had not forgotten to be human beings.

We waited a little while for Rhonda, Dr. Steiner's secretary, to come with my discharge papers and instructions for follow-up, and then we were free to go.

Spending a while in the new world of wondrous, even magical, technology, had indeed been an adventure. We would be telling about it, and remembering it for a long time. And we would be expecting good news from it in six months.

11

Looking Back, Looking Forward

Remembering

It was September 28, 1995. An MRI six months before had indicated that what remained of the tumor at the time of the Gamma Knife radiosurgery had begun to shrink. As we had been told, just as its cells had been slow to grow, they would be slow to die. Now, an MRI I was to have one year after the Gamma Knife was something we looked forward to with great expectancy.

My appointment was at the nearby imaging facility. Probably my confident feeling that there would be a happy outcome to what I was about to undergo led me to think back four and a half years to the spring of 1991.

The recurring ache in the back of my neck had started that January and I truly had thought it wasn't anything more serious than a reaction to stress built up from trying to do too much over the holidays. Then in March came those eerie episodes of disorientation and the feeling I was floating in space when I would get out of the car sometimes. Who knows what would have happened if I hadn't finally been pushed into having an MRI and finding out what was causing obvious signals that something seriously was wrong?

Four and a half years. So many things about them ran through my mind as I waited a few minutes until a nurse came to get me for my session inside the familiar MRI cylinder.

The Friday afternoon telephone call late in June. The shock from hearing those two frightening words: *brain tumor.* The disbelief and the tears that followed. The calm rationalizing later and the resolve to face and take in stride whatever might lie ahead regarding the tumor. That resolve had been shaken, sometimes almost totally broken, at low periods over the years since. Yet, it always had been possible to renew the determination and faith that would bring it back.

Then there was our amazement in looking at MRI images for the first time. I still can see the scary outline of the tumor pressing against the brainstem. From what was explained to us and from what we could see, we realized how difficult and delicate an operation would be. But there had been no question about my having to have one. I thought of my trip to the library to study the brain and brain tumors in the medical encyclopedia. There was no way of knowing then how long my case would continue and how valuable what I learned would be in understanding things that had to be done.

The first operation and the letdown from finding out that despite the long hours of difficult surgery, only part of the tumor had been removed. The disturbing prospect of another operation that had been a cloud hanging over me for a while. I remembered the New Year's Eve resolution that got my mind out from under it. How really frustrated I was, though, with the slow pace of recovery from aftermaths of the operation. It was a good thing I had so much encouragement from so many people.

And I thought of how much we had enjoyed the long respite in 1992 and most of 1993 from any evidence of reborn tumor activity. But then, late in 1993, the ominous growth that was detected in new MRI images. I was terribly stubborn in refusing to accept the reality of it until symptoms of pressure from the growth became so evident and severe that I had no choice.

The two stages of operation in Washington. We had come to realize more and more what a miraculous surgical accomplishment it was to get to and remove so much of the tumor, considering its size and location. With the realization came gratitude that never could be expressed in full measure.

My thoughts turned also to lessons in patience that I had learned at home and from the wonderful staff in Washington. Thanks to them, I discovered how important it is to value every single inch of progress in a recovery that can be painfully slow. For every inch gets you closer to being able to do things that often seem beyond reach.

It was at this point in my reflections that a nurse came and told me they were ready for me. Now I was back to the present. The MRI cylinder was waiting for me. Before long, we would know whether the tumor had been stilled for what we hoped would be forever.

Bright Outlook

My wooden rosary beads were with me for the MRI. They had been my anchor so often that I couldn't conceive of going through an imaging without them. And that certainly was true this time in getting pictures that would show what effect the Gamma Knife had had on the tumor. Seeing favorable results would be just the added lift I needed to keep my spirits high with regard to my recovery progress.

Considering everything, I really had fared remarkably well. I was sorry to have lost most of the hearing in one ear, but I had adjusted to it and didn't think of it as a handicap. The double vision hadn't changed, but I had learned to compensate for it. And I hadn't given up thinking that some morning I could open my eyes and be able to see perfectly through both of them. As for the facial numbness, I had refused to accept it as permanent. Happily, I had detected some feeling coming back, and the numbness had become confined to the area of my cheek.

As far as my swallowing was concerned, it was almost back to normal and I could eat all kinds of food. My weight was reasonably close to what it was supposed to be. And I could walk anywhere without a cane. I did take it with me sometimes, however, just in case I got tired and felt a need for it.

There still were some negatives, I must admit. My memory hadn't come back all the way. Sometimes I would think it had, but then there would be occasions when I would be frustrated and angry with myself for not remembering things I should have been able to think of right away. There had been great improvement, though. And I knew I had to keep working to sharpen my ability to concentrate. My voice had improved, but it was still hoarse at times. And, strangely, it was affected by humidity. In heavy air, I would almost lose it entirely; obviously, this had something to do with the injury to my vocal cord. Another strange thing was a problem I had with crowds. Being in even a slightly crowded area would make me so nervous and confused that I would have to get away from it.

But these problems weren't of great concern to me; I was sure that with time they would be overcome or disappear.

On balance, then, I had much to be thankful for in the physical strides I had made and every reason to be optimistic about further progress. Included in that optimism was full confidence that the MRI I was having on this day would show the Gamma Knife had done what we all hoped it would do.

New Meanings

Exciting news came from Dr. Steiner a few days later regarding the wonderful Gamma Knife. What had remained of the tumor had decreased in size approximately 35 percent. Its cells indeed were dying. Radiosurgery had done its miraculous work. What relief and happiness that report brought us.

There would be another MRI in six months and others at intervals to be determined later. I was sure they would continue to show the tumor had been conquered as a physical presence. Mentally its presence would remain forever inside as a reminder that never again could there be a *really* bad day for me.

Along with strides I had made in recovering from effects that had hit me so hard after the two-stage operation in Washington, I was buoyed by another kind of progress. This involved the promise I had made to myself to take life less for granted and enjoy the gifts it offers every day.

From the beginning, I had felt there was one sure way to go about fulfilling that promise. This was to recapture the enthusiasm and exhilaration of simple things we did, not permitting ever-widening preoccupations, responsibilities, and obligations to engross us and leave no time for little things.

Perhaps I have been a Pollyanna in all this. We grow more "sophisticated" as life becomes more complex and we tend to shut out simple pursuits and satisfactions. But the good feeling and greater appreciation of being alive I have received from what I like to call "revisiting spring" tell me there's nothing wrong with being simplistic about what gives meaning to life.

And, really, it's so satisfying when I think I'm in too much of a rush to stop to "smell the roses" to catch myself and say, "Wait! The beauty and the fragrance may have withered away when you do have time to stop some other day."

My life has taken on added meaning in the satisfaction received from helping other brain-tumor patients with insights gained from my experiences. The word does get around. I've had patients call me from faraway places to ask particular questions. They have heard about me through the doctors and through other patients I met at the medical centers or with whom I have had personal contact since. The help I am able to give them gives me a feeling of gratification that is warm and rewarding.

The importance of such communication is critical. The prevalence of brain tumors has become much more widely publicized since my odyssey began. And it is significant that much of the increased attention has been focused on children.

An example was the cover story in the July 24, 1995 issue of *U.S. News & World Report*. This told of the "medical miracle" of two brainstem tumor operations performed on 7-year-old Matthew Anderson by Dr. Ben Carson, chief of pediatric neurosurgery at Johns Hopkins Hospital in Baltimore. The story detailed how these operations demonstrated why Dr. Carson had become world recognized for his outstanding skill with brain-tumor surgery on children. Nothing could have illustrated more clearly that brain tumors occur at all ages, beginning with the very young. Awareness of this continues to increase.

It is pertinent to my story that this same issue of *U.S. News & World Report* included a rating of America's best hospitals. It was not surprising that such skill as Dr.

Carson's would be present at Johns Hopkins. Along with numerous other specialties, the famous Baltimore institution was ranked as one of the foremost in neurology. Another example of my good fortune is that in writing this book we have had the benefit of highly valued help and advice from one of the fine neurologists there.

Now, as one of two closing notes in this story, it is important to point out that there are organizations active in brain-tumor research and education. I didn't know about them until the time of my surgery in Washington. I'm sure, though, that had I known, I would have gained from communicating with them. That's why I feel it is wise for others who face or have undergone brain-tumor operations to have information on them. They are listed with brief descriptions in the accompanying appendix.

The other closing note is a happy one that came from my next MRI. This was in the spring of 1996. Dr. Steiner's measurement of the remainder of the tumor showed a further reduction. The decrease in size from what it had been before the Gamma Knife radiosurgery was now 40 percent. What a thrill it was to receive this word from Dr. Steiner and Dr. Sekhar.

How beautiful the gift of life has become to me. I am so grateful to God and to all the wonderful individuals along the way who have made it possible for me to keep it and to cherish it as never before.

———————

Appendix

BRAIN TUMOR ORGANIZATIONS

FEDERAL

NIH Neurological Institute
P. O. Box 5801
Bethesda, Maryland 20824
(301) 496-5751 or 1-800-352-9424
Fax: (301) 402-2186

The Institute is a component of the National Institutes of Health. It is the leading federal supporter of research on disorders of the brain and central nervous system. The Institute also sponsors an active public information program and answers questions about diagnosis, treatment, and research related to brain and spinal cord tumors.

PRIVATE

Leading private organizations focusing on brain tumors are members of a network known as the North American Brain Tumor Coalition. The Coalition's purposes are to raise public awareness of brain tumors and their rising incidence, as well as to advocate increased research funding and health care. Other issues affecting brain tumor patients are also addressed.

The following member organizations can be of great help to patients and families in the services rendered:

American Brain Tumor Association
2720 River Road, Suite 146
Des Plaines, Illinois 60018
(847) 827-9910
Patient Line: 1-800-886-2282
Fax: (847) 827-9918

The Association, ABTA for short, provides a variety of services. These include: more than 20 publications addressing brain tumors, their treatment, and coping; nationwide resource listings of support groups and physicians offering investigative treatments; a pen-pal program called *Connections;* and a biennial national symposium for patients and their families. ABTA also funds brain tumor research and publishes *Message Line,* a newsletter issued three times a year.

The Brain Tumor Society
84 Seattle Street
Boston, Massachusetts 02134
(617) 783-0340 or 1-800-770-8287
Fax: (617) 783-9712

The Society raises funds to advance carefully selected scientific research projects and improve clinical care. Its *Color Me Hope Resource Guide* provides information about diagnosis, treatment, resources, and coping.

Heads Up, the Society's quarterly newsletter, has a question and answer column and features pertinent articles. Sponsored education programs include seminars and conferences for researchers and physicians, as well as training for support-group leaders.

The Children's Brain Tumor Foundation
42 Memorial Plaza
Pleasantville, New York 10570
(914) 747-0301
Fax: (914) 747-0381

Established in 1988, the Foundation is active in research, support, and education. Grants are awarded to leading academic medical centers in the region for basic and clinical studies. Patients' families are helped to cope through free monthly support groups for parents, a parent-to-parent network, and funds to cover initial costs of individual counseling for parents by certified specialists. To help parents in dealing with the complexities facing them, a free *Resource Guide* with both technical and practical information is published.

NOTE: Two additional organizations for children and their families provide services in their immediate geographical areas. Activities include promoting public awareness, sponsoring research, publishing educational materials, and furnishing helpful information to families. They are:

Brain Tumor Foundation for Children
2231 Perimeter Park Drive, Suite 9
Atlanta, Georgia 30341
(770) 458-5554
(A member of the Coalition)

Childhood Brain Tumor Foundation
12141 Pineneedle Court
Woodbridge, Virginia 22192
(703) 494-0320
(A relatively new group gradually expanding its work.)

National Brain Tumor Foundation
785 Market Street, Suite 1600
San Francisco, California 94103
(415) 284-0208
Patient services: 1-800-934-CURE
Fax: (415) 284-0209

The Foundation carries out a two-fold mission. Along with funding promising research, it provides help for patients and families in a number of ways. National and regional conferences and seminars it sponsors help to prepare patients for challenges they face. A publication, *Brain Tumors: A Guide*, answers questions for families.

Patient support is provided through a growing national network of organized groups. *Search*, a newsletter published four times a year, updates more than 16,000 families.

Associate Coalition Member
Brain Tumor Foundation of Canada
111 Waterloo Street, Suite 201
London Ontario N6B 2M4
Canada
(519) 642-7755
Fax: (519) 642-7192

This affiliated organization provides services similar to those in the U.S.: research funding, patient and family support activity, publication of pediatric and adult-patient resource guides, issuance of a quarterly newsletter, *BrainStorm*.

A Special Function
National Familial Brain Tumor Registry
The Johns Hopkins Oncology Center
600 North Wolfe Street
Baltimore, Maryland 21287-8936
(410) 955-0227

The Registry collects information from families with two or more members affected by a primary malignant brain tumor. This agency hopes to gain insights on potential genetic and environmental sources of brain tumors.